What Dumbass Doctors Tell You

A Patient's Perspective

Dr. Theresa Errante-Parrino

WHAT DUMBASS DOCTORS TELL YOU: A PATIENT'S PERSPECTIVE

1405 SW 6th Avenue • Ocala, Florida 34471 • Phone 352-622-1825 • Fax 352-622-1875
Website: www.atlantic-pub.com • Email: sales@atlantic-pub.com
SAN Number: 268-1250

Library of Congress Control Number: 2020911057

Printed in the United States

PROJECT MANAGER: Jessie Ranew
INTERIOR LAYOUT AND JACKET DESIGN: Nicole Sturk

DEDICATION

I dedicate this book to my mother, Maria, for her loving support and for encouraging me to write this book; to my brother, Anthony, for the support you have provided to me; to the rest of my family and friends for the love, understanding, and support that you have always given me.

AUTHOR'S NOTE

This is a work of nonfiction. Some names and identifying information have been changed to keep the identity and privacy of persons and facilities confidential.

Table of Contents

Preface

This book is based on my experiences with what I heard from dumbass doctors when I started my journey with breast cancer. I feel obligated to share what they told me and what I actually found to be true based on my own experience and research, so that you don't fall into the same trap I did.

If you have some type of concern, don't brush it off and say, "I'm sure it's nothing." Be persistent, seek out new doctors, do your research, and get it checked out with second or even third opinions. But most importantly, know that it is okay to ask questions of your doctors. Be your own advocate—it may save your life.

CHAPTER 1

My Story

Grandma had inflammatory breast cancer and died at age 60. Mom started her cancer journey at age 40 with breast cancer, known as ductal carcinoma in situ (DCIS), which returned four years after she had undergone chemo, radiation, surgery, and hormone blockers. She developed skin cancer a few years later, which also came back. After the second skin cancer surgery, she was fine for eight years. Then she was diagnosed with lung cancer. Actually, she was misdiagnosed for five years.

She had never smoked anything, but the doctor said she'd developed it from dad's secondhand smoke. Dad had prostate cancer, as well as stomach cancer, which metastasized to liver cancer. He died at age 70 from cancer metastasis. With all this in mind, I just naturally assumed that one day I too would develop cancer. I figured I was doomed by genetics, and I was right.

I was diagnosed in June of 2016 at age 41 with Stage III-C breast cancer—invasive ductal carcinoma with metastasis to axillary lymph nodes and 11 out of 16 positive lymph nodes. I underwent chemotherapy treatment for six months but was diagnosed with the same Stage III-C breast cancer at age 44 in February 2019.

It all started out with a sporadic sharp pain in my upper right arm that became eventually more aggressive and frequent. At first, I thought it was just a sprained muscle or some type of trauma to the arm, but after about three months of increasing pain and frequency, it was time for a doctor's visit.

In the second month, I noticed a small breast lump as well, and started to panic. I mentioned it to my mom and my friend Elizabeth. I told them that I would be going to the doctor to get it checked out because I thought I might have breast cancer.

Of course, Mom just said, "Don't worry about it—it's most likely nothing. You don't have cancer."

Elizabeth said: "Just go and get it checked and wait for the results."

They both thought I was overreacting—jumping to conclusions, being a hypochondriac, and getting all worked up over nothing.

"Fine," I said, but I still thought I had cancer. I quickly learned to drop the conversation about the c-word with them. They didn't want to hear it. No one ever wants to hear, "You have cancer," but I was realistic. I played the "what if" game in my head. *What if this* is *something serious? What if I do have cancer?*

I went to a breast surgeon just to be sure. I mentioned that I had a pain in my upper arm and felt a small lump in my breast, explaining my family history.

Yes, I know I have a strong probability of getting breast cancer, as my grandma and mom had it. They wanted me to be prepared, but I expected the worst already.

In the meantime, the doctor ordered a mammogram. The doctor told me that it most likely was nothing but would order the test just as a precautionary measure. I asked about my arm pain, and he said, again: "I doubt it's anything. I'll give you a two-week follow-up appointment to review your mammogram."

At the follow-up appointment, the mammogram results showed a 15x5-millimeter mass in the outer right breast area where I'd felt the lump. The next step was to have a biopsy to determine what the mass was. Again, my anxiety got the better of me, and thoughts of cancer consumed me. It was definitely something I didn't want to think about, but there it was in my head. My arm pain continued as well. In addition to everything else, now I also had the anxiety of waiting for the biopsy results. What was I supposed to think about?

Two weeks later, I was back at the doctor's with my mom for the biopsy results. It was a mammary lipoma—nothing to worry about, I was told. It was a noncancerous bit of fatty tissue that would go away without treatment. What a relief! Not cancer.

Over the course of about two months, though, I felt that the lipoma was getting bigger, so I went back to the doctor. I explained that there was something more going on: The lump was becoming more prominent, and my arm pain was getting worse. The doctor reassured me that it was just the noncancerous fatty tissue lipoma. I had my doubts, so to be safe—and to cover his butt—the doctor ordered a magnetic resonance imaging (MRI) scan and a genetic blood test (MYvantage Genetic Test) to assess my breast cancer risk.

I thought, *Wow, this doctor is great! He is thorough and wants to check me out. Finally, with some convincing, he's listening to me and taking me seriously.*

There was something on the MRI. But what was the something? Everything was negative for cancer up to this point, so what could it be? Was my intuition correct? Was I really doomed? Was it breast cancer? If so, how bad was it? What type of breast cancer did I have? What size was it? How aggressive was it? I took my speculations to Google.

I researched and decided on two potential diagnoses: ductal carcinoma in situ, or DCIS (cancer contained within the ducts), or invasive ductal carcinoma (cancer spread beyond the ducts).

The MRI results showed what was now an 18-millimeter area of clumped enhancement at the 8:30 position and a 12-millimeter enhancement of the side and lower area of the breast, just above where I'd felt the lump.

"Oh no," I thought. "Here we go again." My initial biopsy from two months prior was still healing, and now it was time for a second biopsy.

Again, trying not to dwell on the thought that I might have cancer, mom and I went in for the follow-up visit to get the results of the second biopsy. I had warned my mom just a few days before the appointment, saying: "Don't be surprised if the results are cancer."

Again, she replied, "Stop it! Think positive!" It drove me crazy. Thinking positive had nothing to do with the fact that I might have cancer. If I had cancer, I had cancer. Yes, a positive attitude can help ease some of the physical effects of having cancer, but it didn't change the fact that I could still have cancer.

When the doctor entered the room with a nurse, I knew immediately that the results were going to be bad. From my background in the medical field, I knew that there is an extra person in the room to serve as a witness when bad news is delivered to a patient.

"You have cancer." I think that even the doctor was surprised by the diagnosis.

The biopsy results showed a 2.1-centimeter, Grade 2 invasive ductal carcinoma (IDC), which was estrogen receptor (ER) positive at 100 percent, progesterone receptor (PR) positive at 100 percent, and human epidermal growth factor receptor 2 (HER-2) negative.

Lucky for me, the doctor said, I had a "good" cancer. *What the hell does that mean? How can cancer be good? It is the "big c"—cancer!* At my look of agitation, he went on to explain that the type of cancer I had has responded well to surgery, chemotherapy, radiation therapy, and hormone therapy in other cases. So, it was a good cancer.

I'd been right—I *did* have cancer. Mom was in a state of shock and disbelief. As for me, this hadn't come as too much of a surprise. I'd had my suspicions from the very start of the arm pain more than four months earlier.

I was somewhat mentally prepared. I didn't even shed a tear when given the diagnosis. Google had helped me narrow it down, and I was leaning more toward the "in situ" findings myself, so I hadn't thought it would be so invasive already. I started asking questions of the doctor, and it obviously shocked him how I was handling the news. I had warned mom, but she still didn't want to hear it. So much for thinking positive!

I was a young, single medical professional working 50 to 60 hours a week. I held both supervisory and teaching positions at a state college. But now I was faced with the diagnosis of breast cancer, wondering about surgical treatment options—lumpectomy, mastectomy, double mastectomy, reconstruction, implants, plastic surgery, and working or not working?

If I stopped working, there was no telling how my diagnosis would affect me financially. Fortunately, it was June, and I had the summer off. I would be returning to work in August for the fall semester but wound up submitting Family and Medical Leave Act (FMLA) paperwork for November 2016 under doctor's orders. This allowed me to have surgery during Thanksgiving break, recover over the winter break, and return to work in January of the following year.

Regarding the decision of what type of surgery to undergo, I was told that either a lumpectomy or mastectomy would be appropriate. With a lumpectomy, the chance of recurrence was slightly higher than with a mastectomy. The mastectomy would take all the tissue, and there would be no chance of recurrence. If I chose mastectomy, I could have a single mastectomy, which would leave me with one breast and uneven, or I could opt for a double mastectomy—both would require reconstruction and plastic surgery. The double mastectomy was recommended if I wanted to have "breasts." I was big-breasted as it was, at a natural 36DD.

I decided to go with the bilateral mastectomy, eliminating my chances of recurrence. I'd get new, smaller boobs, look lifted and perky, be even on both sides, and all would be great. I asked the breast surgeon if the breast implants could be done at the same time as the surgery and was assured that this could be done. The breast surgeon would team up with the plastics and reconstructive surgeon on the day of the surgery, and all could be done in one surgery and in one day. I double-checked with the plastics guy just to be sure.

Searching for a plastic surgeon with reconstructive knowledge was another challenge. For the first consult, I took mom with me to the physician recommended by the breast surgeon. The office was located in the same building as the breast surgeon, which made it easy and convenient. It was an all-glass building that sat on the waterfront of the Intracoastal Waterway. It had a beautiful waiting room and a friendly front-office staff. When my name was called, mom and I walked into the exam room. The nurse asked me to change into a gown and wait on the exam table. Mom took a seat in the corner chair of the exam room.

An older gentleman doctor came in and asked why I was there.

I said, "For a consult for reconstruction after mastectomy."

The doctor did an exam, took measurements, and explained that he would not reconstruct at the same time of the surgery but six to nine months later. He also stated that I would need tissue expanders for six months after healing before he could place implants.

He came back to me again and began playing with my boobs, stating that he needed to get a feel for the weight of each one. He seemed to me to enjoy himself a bit too much. I pulled back, and even mom said something to him as a distraction. Yes, I got felt up by a doctor in front of my mother in the doctor's office. I'd had enough of that, so I got dressed and didn't even stop at the checkout desk on the way out. Mom and I left, saying, "Time for another doctor!"

The second consult was with a younger reconstructive plastic surgeon on the other side of town. Again, the office was in a new building in a nice location and boasted a cute doctor. Mom came with me to this appointment as well. We pretended that I hadn't seen Dr. Feel Me Up. We were just starting over with a new doctor.

I asked the same questions: Can we do reconstruction and implants during the double mastectomy? Yes. Can you tag team with the breast surgeon? Yes. Do I need to have tissue expanders? No. Just what I wanted to hear.

He provided me some options on the sizes and types of implants I could choose from—saline, silicone, or new gel "gummy bear" material. He also asked me what type of profile I wanted: low or high. He tossed me samples of the different types to feel, play with, and decide. I caught and tossed these samples to mom. We started to play catch with the sample gel breast implants. I decided on the gel high-profile 700-cubic centimeter implants, a "D" cup. It was a size smaller than my natural size, but that was okay by me.

Mom and I decided to go ahead with this doctor since he'd said everything I wanted to hear. He had a great bedside manner and came recommended not only by the breast surgeon but also by my neighbor. Surgery was to be coordinated between him and the breast surgeon.

During this time, life went on. Dad was also diagnosed with stomach cancer, which metastasized to his liver. He had just finished chemotherapy and was now undergoing radiation therapy. Over the past few months, I had seen firsthand what a cancer patient goes through. I saw how draining treatments were—how dad had no energy; how he lost his hair from chemo; how tired he was from radiation; how he just wanted to sit, relax, and watch TV, and not be bothered with the stresses of life. Dad didn't even know how bad my cancer was or what decisions I was making regarding my own health. My mom was there for me and had to deal with two family members going through cancer at the same time. Oh, my poor mom—the strength she had to have to deal with her husband nearing the end of this battle and her daughter just beginning hers.

My neighbor was diagnosed with breast cancer in June as well. She underwent a bilateral mastectomy and opted for reconstruction. She had a different breast surgeon than I did, but we both used the same plastic surgeon for reconstruction. She was happy with her outcome and would undergo reconstruction in a few weeks. She had the surgery and had to wait for the skin to stretch with breast expanders before getting implants put in. She did not need any other treatment besides surgery. We compared notes and bonded over our cancer.

November 21, 2016 was surgery day. Nervous, anxious, and gowned up, I was ready for my bilateral mastectomy with immediate implant reconstruction. The doctor came in to mark me up, explained the procedure, and informed me he would test axillary lymph nodes during the surgery to ensure that the cancer hadn't spread.

"Don't worry," he said. "I doubt anything will be positive." He explained that the surgery would take about four hours from start to finish. Once the surgery was finished, I would wake up in the hospital for an overnight stay.

Okay, I was prepared for this. Time to go to the operating room.

I woke up in the hospital room, all bandaged up. I felt my chest, and yes, I had boobs. I slept through the night, and when I woke in the morning, the breast surgeon came to visit. He told me that the four-hour surgery had ended up lasting eight hours, and he'd had to call in a third doctor to help with the case because the cancer was worse than expected. He told me that 11 out of 16 lymph nodes were positive for cancer, which might have been the reason for my arm pain. The surgeon was shocked at having gone from a "nothing-to-worry-about" cancer case to a far worse situation of metastases.

Now that the lymph nodes were positive, the entire situation had changed. Further testing and aggressive treatment options had to be explored. Having positive lymph nodes means that the cancer can spread anywhere in the body through the circulation. If this happens, the cancer can return, or spread to a different part of the body. It was time to go cancer hunting. An eyes-to-thighs positron emission tomography (PET) scan was ordered for three weeks out, to give me time to heal, have the drains removed, and follow up with the surgeon and plastics team.

The next day, I was discharged from the hospital and got to go home. This was quite a task. I had drains hanging down both sides of my chest; I was in some pain, and I was toting paperwork for home health. Mom got me home and set up in bed before going to her house to stay with my dad, who was becoming progressively worse. I told her to just stay with dad. I'd have the nurse come do measurements and clean out my drains.

All was well until the nurse came the following day to do my drains. That was a disaster. First, it seemed as if she wasn't trained on how to strip the tubes, or maybe she just didn't want to. I explained to her how to do it, but she was of no help, so I fired her right then and there. I had to call mom and ask her to come and do them. I didn't want to have dad left alone for too long, but I didn't have a choice. I called the neighbor to see if she could come to help me the next day. She told me that she was going back in for surgery to get her boobs and couldn't come. Mom would have to come again, and then it would be up to me to do them myself.

After a week, it was time for follow-up. The plastics doctor took out the drains, took a look, and said that everything was healing well and that I could go home. I was thrilled.

Just two days later, though, my sutures began to reopen. I called the plastics guy, and he said that the skin was stretched tight, but that the sutures had been in for a week, so the skin was closed. "Don't worry. If anything else happens, call me back."

On December 9, 2016—PET scan day—I was changing into a gown when I noticed that my incision line was leaking. More sutures had opened, and the wound was oozing. I told the tech, and she called the plastics doctor. I needed the scan, so the tech and I covered the incision with gauze and tape and proceeded with the scan.

After I was done, I drove over to the doctor's office to have him look at the now-open incision. Right there in the procedure room, he sutured me up again. I thought it was a bit strange to have sutures put in at the office, but it was convenient, and it needed to get done. I was told to keep an eye on it, and if anything happened, I was to it to call the office or his cell phone. *Wow! A doctor actually gave out his personal cell number! That about never happens.*

Two days later, on the weekend (of course), I noticed that the wound was opening again, and the area was red and hot. I saw a small black area on the incision line that was now exposed. It was obviously time to use that cell phone number. The doctor told me to go to the local emergency room, and he would meet me there. I was told just to ask for him and not sign in. Wow, preferential treatment!

On my way there, I picked up mom and took her with me. I had a feeling I could be admitted or perhaps even need to go into surgery to have the implant removed. When we arrived at the ER, I gave my name and asked for the doctor. Mom and I were taken directly into a procedure room, and I was asked to change into a gown. *Here we go again.*

The doctor took a look and said that I needed to be re-stitched. The doctor asked mom if she was squeamish, and when she said no, he said that she would be the assistant. Again, I thought this was odd. Why was my mom the assistant? The ER nurse did bring us supplies, but that was it. The doctor put in about 21 new sutures to close the open wound. When the procedure was complete, he gave me a prescription for antibiotics. This was exactly how I'd wanted to spend my Saturday night.

Later on, I gave some thought to the situation. I realized that the entire ER hospital visit was a cover-up, and that is what I still think to this day. There was no documentation that I was there because I hadn't signed into the ER. There had been no nurse helping so, again, no documentation. There was no bill, no copay, no charges submitted to insurance, no nothing. *Hmm, something is not right. Why wouldn't anything be documented?* As anyone in healthcare knows: If it wasn't documented, it wasn't done. At least the wound was closed, not oozing anymore.

—

At the follow-up appointment at the breast surgeon's office, mom and I anxiously waited for the doctor to enter the room with the PET scan results. Upon review, they showed that my right infraclavicular lymph node was now also infected with cancer, and treatment had to be aggressive. The cancer had already spread from my breast to the axillary lymph nodes, and now another lymph node in my upper chest just below my clavicle was infected. I'd already had a bilateral mastectomy, but I still had cancer. I was given a referral to a medical oncologist to discuss chemotherapy. These results were not what I'd wanted to hear. Dad had only just finished his chemotherapy a few months before, and now it was my turn.

—

About five days after I'd had the sutures redone, I was back in the emergency room, though at a different hospital. The wound had reopened, the black spot was getting bigger, and now I had a fever. After the ER doctor examined me, he said that I had implant exposure, and they had to come out. The removal of the implants needed to be pushed a week out, so they could treat my fever and infection. It was also Christmas week, so the doctor and operating room (OR) couldn't accommodate me.

During my three-day hospital stay for infection, I experienced a reaction to vancomycin—one of the strongest antibiotics there is. I got what they call "red man syndrome." It is not a true allergy, but a reaction that occurs when the vancomycin is running too fast in the IV, and your face and arms get all red and itchy. Now comes all the medication for the allergic reaction. Would it never end? Surgery for the implant removal was scheduled for December 28, with the same plastic surgeon who'd put them in and had re-sutured me.

This gave my mom a few days to make arrangements for my dad. It was bad enough that she would leave him for an hour to visit me in the hospital during my three-day stay, but she couldn't leave him home alone for the hours it'd take while I had my surgery. She had to drive me to the procedure, drive me home from the procedure, and stay with me for a day to ensure that I was okay—typical surgical protocol. She had no other choice but to put him into the Respite Care Program of Hospice. This was a five-day program where he would go to Hospice house, have a private room, be supervised and managed for his stomach cancer, and would come home in five days. Perfect: Dad would be taken care of, and mom could tend to my needs while still visiting dad in Hospice as well.

After dad had been in Hospice for three days, he took a turn for the worse. Mom told me that I should go see him. I was only three days post-op myself, but when I got there, I knew mom had been right. Dad was medicated and nonverbal, lying in the fetal position with his eyes glazed over. He was pale and lifeless, though he moaned every now and again. I talked to him just a bit but couldn't look at him.

When the nurse came in, I asked her some questions. She said that dad could still hear, so she pulled me outside to answer my questions. After this conversation, I went back into dad's room to say my goodbyes. I knew this would be the last time I would see him alive. I don't know how my mom went every day for the next two weeks to visit with him. I couldn't go back. However, I couldn't help but wonder: If I hadn't had surgery and he didn't go into Respite, would he have lived longer? Would he have been more comfortable at home?

—

My medical oncology appointment was on January 4, 2017. I sort of knew what to expect from treatment since my dad had just gone through it. I heard that the doctor treated "aggressively," and that was good for my case. I was told that I would need to have chemotherapy and weekly blood tests to monitor the effects of the chemo. As the doctor explained how the schedule worked, I asked her a question and was told to hold all my questions to the end. *Um, what?* It was like she had her spiel memorized and couldn't be distracted, or she would need to start over. I waited and tried to remember the questions I had as she went through her monologue. She rubbed me the wrong way.

She also told me that I was not allowed to work—she would sign the Family and Medical Leave Act (FMLA) papers, but I couldn't work. My career was just starting to take off, and now I was being told that I couldn't work. How was I supposed to pay for all these medical bills? But, of course, it wasn't her problem; it was my problem. FMLA "secured" my position with the intent of me returning to work. In the meantime, I could have all my procedures and focus on getting well. I had health insurance through my employer, so no need to worry about medical expenses.

The doctor told me I would have chemo treatments once a week for eight weeks in the office and have my blood drawn at the same time. She also stated that I would need to have a port put in, through which the chemo could be delivered. Oh, great—another surgery. My port surgery was scheduled for two weeks out and would be done by the breast surgeon. I didn't want to have the chemo but was convinced to take it. Once a week for eight weeks didn't seem that difficult. I could do it.

—

The day of my port surgery arrived. It was no big deal—an outpatient procedure with no complications. I started chemo the next day. The area was sore, but access was good.

The first day of chemo was not too bad. What I didn't like was that I was sitting in a big, open room with other cancer patients who were all hooked up to IVs as well. It was very depressing, and it was the first time that I felt like a cancer patient. Since it was my first time, I was given a congratulatory goodie bag. *Really? Congrats, you have cancer. Here is a goodie bag!* The tote bag actually had some good things in it, though. There was a blanket, a coffee gift card, tissues, colored pencils, a word search, coloring book, snacks, and bottled water.

When I asked how long the treatment would take, I didn't expect to hear four hours. There were pre-meds (anti-nausea, anti-diarrhea, antihistamine), then the chemo, then fluids. The only good thing was that since it was my first day of chemo, mom was able to sit next to me. After this, she had to stay in the waiting room.

When the day was over and I went to check out, the woman said, "See you tomorrow!"

I explained that I only get chemo once a week.

She said, "Tomorrow is a fluid day."

Fluid day? What is that? What happened to once-a-week chemo?

Fluid day is two to three hours of just fluid and follows chemo day every week. So now we were up to two days a week of appointments . . . or so I thought. Apparently, there was a *third day*. After fluid day came shot day. But shot day wasn't just shot day. It was shot *and* fluid day. The shot was to help boost immunity and stimulate blood cell production. Terrible bone pain followed shot day and lasted three days. My diet consisted of Tylenol and Gatorade following the shot. No one ever told me all this. If I'd known all this beforehand, I would not have agreed. Who wants to hear you will be sick for six out of seven days a week? On day seven, I'd start to feel better, only to go through it all again the next day. So much for the once-a-week chemo!

—

On January 25, 2017, we lost dad to stomach and liver cancer after a two-year fight. This was not easy. I had been on chemo for two weeks and was starting to have side effects—constant nausea, fatigue, thinning hair, and immuno-incompetence. I wasn't supposed to be around people, which was hard. I had to wear a face mask while giving dad's eulogy at his wake.

I had seen what cancer had done to him, and I hoped that I, too, wouldn't end up lying in a casket in a few months. Mom was in distress about this too. How could she lose a husband and a daughter in the same year? I couldn't do that to her. I had to recover. So, I proceeded with chemo over the next few months.

Yes, months. When I finished the first eight weeks of chemo and thought it was my last day, it wasn't. It was the end of the first chemo *drug*. Then came the start of 12 weeks with a second chemo drug, still on the same "one-day-a-week" schedule, which was actually six days a week. By this time, I'd lost my hair and my appetite. I felt fatigued and had no energy; I was immunocompromised, had become anemic, and was isolated. I couldn't have visitors, couldn't go out (except for chemo), couldn't be around children, and couldn't work. I had three more months of chemo treatments with weekly blood tests and doctor visits.

I finally completed chemo on May 9, 2017. This was followed by a PET scan to ensure that there were no "hot spots" in my body and that the chemo had done its job. Finally, some positive news: I had a negative PET scan. No hot spots! The chemo worked, and I was cancer free! Since the chemo was finished, the next step was getting the port removed. It was uncomfortable, and I preferred to not have foreign objects in my body. I was also anxious to take off the "port awareness bracelet" that I'd worn from the very first day.

I was also allowed to go back to work. Hooray! I'd been on FMLA for a year. I felt very fortunate that my position had been held for that long. I was able to use all my sick leave, personal time, time from the sick-leave pool, and short-term disability, and was granted administrative leave. I'd exhausted every option to keep my position on hold. I worked reduced hours that summer, so that I could ease back into my full-time role. It worked out well because I was able to work around my doctor appointments.

The next step was to get some boobs! I had been flat-chested for six months after the first set had to come out due to the infection and implant exposure. I found a new plastic and cosmetic doctor who was willing to give me breasts. I knew the profile, type, and size I wanted, so the process was a bit easier this time. Surgery was scheduled for June 9, 2017.

The doctor recommended that I not get the 700 cc implants (size D) since I'd had so many complications previously. Instead I chose the 500 cc implants (size C) this time. This surgeon, a middle-aged man, who had more experience with cases like mine, made all the difference. I felt very comfortable with him and had no hesitation. This time, I was up and about in three days and had no problems with the implants, sutures, or anything else. I looked like a C cup, but when I went bra shopping, I barely filled an A cup. That was fine with me. I had boobs, and they were even!

The next few months of healing were a process. Every week, the implants would change a bit. They would soften as the swelling went down, settle as scar tissue grew around them, and feel lighter on my chest, and they took on a more natural shape and feel. I checked in every month with the new plastics doctor and the original breast surgeon to ensure proper healing and to make sure that no further complications arose. Though summer was here again, the pool and beach were off-limits for proper healing.

—

November 16, 2017 started my second year as a cancer patient. I'd had a rough summer with all the changes my body went through with cancer, chemo, implants, re-suturing, implant removal, implants reinsertion, and healing.

I went back and forth to the medical oncologist, breast surgeon, and plastic surgeon every month, but I still had some swelling.

Is this normal? Why is my arm starting to hurt again? Oh no . . . don't tell me I have cancer again, I thought to myself. *How can this be? I just finished chemo five months ago and had a negative PET scan! Am I overthinking this?*

When I mentioned to the breast surgeon that I still had some swelling, he ordered an ultrasound for November 29, 2017. Of course, with the Thanksgiving holiday approaching, I would need to wait a few weeks for a follow-up appointment for the results. There is nothing like trying to get a doctor's appointment scheduled between Thanksgiving and Christmas.

I got my ultrasound results on December 20, 2017. Results stated "swelling," and recommended a repeat ultrasound in three months. Okay, well that meant I was still healing, right? Let's hope.

In January 2018, I was finally cleared to work full time. Since it had been two years since I went on sick leave, my position was given to one of my friends and coworkers. I was reassigned to work in three different departments on the same day for 12 hours a day, five days a week. I was a salaried worker, but this was the assignment. It was a paycheck, so I did it. I was no longer in a supervisory position, so that was a nice change, but the hours were long! I still had to take off some days for follow-up visits and breast pain. Of course, that didn't go over so well with management.

On March 9, 2018, I lost my job due to extended medical leave and continued cancer care. I had to go on Consolidated Omnibus Budget Reconciliation Act (COBRA) benefits for medical coverage, which cost $800 a month! I had no choice. What was I supposed to do, not have medical coverage? That was not going to happen. I'd incurred more than $500,000 in debt with the bilateral mastectomy as it was. I was still having breast issues, still having follow-up appointments, and still having blood work.

———

Three months passed, and the time came for my repeat ultrasound, which was great because I was still having issues with swelling. I'd had the implants for 10 months, and I should have been done healing by now. Since this was about my third ultrasound, I knew what to expect—have the exam, clean up, get dressed, leave, and follow-up with the doctor in two weeks.

My results were the same as three months before: swelling, repeat in three months. *What the heck is going on? Why, I am not healing? There was nothing else to do except to wait another three months.*

CHAPTER 2

Starting Over: Here We Go Again

Two months after my ultrasound, I felt a lump in my right breast, just in the scar line. I called the doctor and asked what should I do, explaining that my arm pain was back, too.

He said that I had another ultrasound scheduled the next month but said not to worry about it, it was most likely scar tissue. I'd had plenty of experience with my boobs—this was not scar tissue. If it were, why would it have taken two and a half years to form? This doctor had been pretty good and aggressive with the treatment, so I decided that I would try not to worry about it, and I'd wait for the ultrasound.

The results came back from the ultrasound, and this time it showed a small area of concern, 5 millimeters with irregular margins. Again I was told that it was most likely scar tissue. Well, with my medical education, I knew that areas of concern with irregular margins are usually suspicious and turn out to be more serious. I asked the doctor to do a biopsy to make sure that it was nothing.

My next appointment was on December 4, 2018, for an in-office surgery, so the doctor could remove what he insisted was "scar tissue." When I was on the table, I asked if he could please go wide and deep enough to ensure that he get all the "scar tissue." I was again told: "Don't worry about it—it's most likely just scar tissue."

Why would the doctor say that without knowing for certain if it were scar tissue or not? Why would the breast surgeon not take me seriously after all the complications I'd had? Why not say: "Well, let's see what the results are before we make any final decisions"? Was it because he was the doctor and wanted to be right? What if he was wrong? What if this was serious? What if it was cancer again?

He cut out my area of concern with the strong conviction that everything was removed, telling me to come back in two weeks for the results.

I went in on December 19, 2018, to get the test results from my "scar tissue" removal. The doctor entered the exam room and said that it was recurrence. I'd had the inkling that something was not right. I'd somehow known that it was not scar tissue but a hard, pea-sized lump.

Oh, great . . . a positive cancer diagnosis . . . again. Merry Christmas to me! Now I had to schedule a PET scan to see if I had cancer anywhere else in my body. My PET scan was scheduled for ten days out, on December 28, 2018. Not only did I have cancer again, but now it was Stage III-C, only one step away from terminal.

A follow-up appointment was scheduled for two weeks out to get my PET scan results.

On January 8, I went back to see the breast surgeon for the results, and they were not good: I had a positive lymph node just under my collarbone on the right side. The doctor told me that he didn't operate on that lymph node, but chemo and radiation would destroy it.

Wait. Hold up. Did he say chemo and radiation? Nope! Not again.

I wanted to go to a specialty cancer treatment center; I wanted a second opinion; I wanted doctors who treated special cases, who have had patients with complications, and who take their patients seriously, without dismissing them. He told me that the closest facility was four hours away, in Tampa, Florida. It was either that or go to Texas. I chose Tampa.

The cancer center called and told me that they had a waiting list, and it would take some time to get in. I said that was okay. I was expecting a three- to five-month wait, but it turned out to be only three weeks. My appointment was set for Friday, February 1, 2019, the day before my 44th birthday.

I had never seen a place like the cancer center before. It had a pharmacy, an art center, a quiet room, a café, and several waiting rooms, all with coffee, tea, a library, and hot chocolate for free; there were charging stations and volunteers who asked if you needed a warm blanket or pillow. *Wow, impressive!* After check-in, they provide each patient with a beeper that tells them where to go.

I had two appointments that day—one with a medical oncologist and the other with a breast surgeon. The medical oncologist had done his homework; He came into the room with four pieces of paper with notes to review with me. He knew my history, complications, treatments—everything. He gave me options, let me ask questions, and took a full hour with me, and he didn't seem rushed. I felt a bit rushed myself, knowing that I had a second appointment, and I didn't want to be late.

He said, "Don't worry. They know you are with me. They will see you when you get to that department. The doctors here work in teams, and they present new cases to a board, so everyone is well informed, and they discuss each case fully prior to talking to the patient."

It was impressive. This oncologist was a relatively young physician at the top of his game. I was impressed. Finally, I had a doctor who listened, took my concerns seriously, and let me ask questions off the cuff.

The breast surgeon was a young female physician who also seemed to know a lot about my case. When she asked me if I'd had a breast MRI recently, I told her no. She asked if I could stay the weekend in Tampa and have an MRI on Monday at 8 a.m. Keep in mind that this was Friday at 2 p.m. What kind of place was this that you could order so late in the day and get an early appointment the next working day? Why had I been waiting three months for diagnostic testing appointments where I lived? I was so impressed with this place. Of course I agreed to stay the weekend and have an MRI Monday at 8 a.m.

On Monday morning, it was the same thing: check-in, registration, pager, and offers of warm blankets and pillows. I had to go to the MRI department that day, but first, I had to go to the IV department to have an IV started for contrast media. Even that department was impressive: They had heating pads to warm your veins, vein-finder lights, fancy technology, and nurses and a phlebotomist who knew what they were doing.

Next, I went to the changing room for MRI. Before the entryway into the room, there was a scanner to check for metal in and on your body—I'd never seen that anywhere before. The MRI tech explained everything step-by-step and tried to ensure my comfort, as well.

The scan took about an hour, and she told me the results would be in the next day. Again, I had been waiting two weeks for test results at home, but here I'd get them the next day? Plus, I was told that the doctor would call me herself with the result, and not the nurse or medical assistant.

Now, after spending the weekend in Tampa, it was time for the four-hour drive home to await the next day's call. The car conversation was about how my mom and I were both so impressed with this facility. The employees were all so kind, caring, and attentive. The doctors were well educated, had tons of technology, and were able to schedule tests from a few hours to just a few days out and have the results within 24 hours.

Now, why did I wait so long to come here? If I'd started here two years ago at the start of my cancer diagnosis, would I have had so many complications?

When I got home, I looked up this specialty cancer center online and found that it was ranked number eight in the country for cancer care, with the Texas facility ranked at number one. I couldn't imagine what it would be like there, if I was so impressed with number eight!

The call came at 11 a.m. on February 5, 2019. The breast surgeon herself was on the phone with my MRI results.

I had been prepared to hear that the cancer had returned but not that I had multiple suspicious areas throughout the region of my right breast. If the local doctor had listened to me about the lump in the first place and ordered an MRI right then, I may not have been in this position. His "don't worry about it" attitude had given me another month's worth of growth.

The specialty doctor wanted to see me again in two weeks to show me the MRI pictures and do the preop exam. She said the MRI pictures were "impressive," and I would need surgery to have these multiple areas removed.

"Impressive"? What does that mean? I would have to wait the two weeks to find out.

She went ahead and scheduled surgery for March 6, only a month away. Another fast turnaround.

On February 21, 2019, I returned to Tampa with my mom for the follow-up visit with the breast surgeon to review my "impressive" MRI and to have my preop appointment.

The MRI showed about seven or eight additional tumors. The doctor explained that it was a good thing I hadn't waited any longer, as my condition was pretty serious. Much of the original breast tissue was still in place, which should have been previously removed with the bilateral mastectomy. *Did the local doctor screw up? Was it too much for him to do? He had two other doctors with him on my case—what roles did they play?* Of course, this doctor couldn't answer any of those questions for me but strongly recommended a redo mastectomy.

I couldn't believe it. I had been cancer-free for only five months, and now I was starting over again. The anxiety was building. *Did I have to do chemo again? Did I need another port? How about radiation? What is my recovery time?*

I was reassured that this redo mastectomy would be done correctly. I would have to see the medical oncologist in Tampa again to see what the post-surgery recommendation would be regarding chemo, radiation, and so on. That appointment would not happen until the pathology report from surgery came back, though. I was also told that the lymph node under my collarbone would be removed as well, and that it was "contaminated."

"You can take that one out?" I asked. I had been told no previously.

The doctor said, "Yes, we take them out. Why take the chance leaving cancer in your body?"

So apparently nothing had been done correctly before.

March 6, 2019, was surgery day. Here I go again. This time it was in a new hospital, with a new set of doctors, and I knew what to expect. My anxiety was running high, so I asked for some "happy juice" (anti-anxiety medication) while I was in preop holding, just to take the edge off before surgery. The doctor came in to mark me up, and off to surgery I went. This two-hour surgery turned into a four-hour surgery, and additional doctors had to be called into the operating room as well. Couldn't anything ever go according to plan?

When I woke up post-op, the doctor told me that some of the nodules were under my right breast implant, and the only way to get to them was to remove the implant. *Oh no, not the implant! After all I had gone through previously, now the implant was removed?* In addition, the lymph node near the collarbone was complex, and a vascular surgeon had to be called in to help. This node had attached itself to the subclavian and brachial arteries—hence my arm pain. The lymph node infringed on the blood supply in my arm, which is why my arm hurt so bad—no oxygen! Good thing mom was there as well; I'm not sure I would have remembered all this as I was coming out of anesthesia.

From there, I was transferred to the medical surgical floor and would be there for three days for recovery. The nice thing was that Moffitt allowed my mom to stay in my room and even brought in a cot for her to sleep on. It was great having here there; I felt like I didn't have to do this alone. I had all-day company.

Mom, however, didn't have such a good time. She said her cot was lumpy, and she was awakened every time the nurses came in to check on me, which even I thought was a lot. I have to say that mom was able to come and go as she pleased; she walked the halls, had access to a fully stocked kitchen, and could help herself to what she wanted whenever. I was able to see the area on the second day of my stay, as I was able to get out of bed and walk around. I thought this kitchen was amazing. The cupboards were stocked with all types of soups, snacks, and paper goods. There was a fridge stocked with all types of juices and sodas, and a freezer full of frozen meals, ice pops, and ice cream. A microwave and coffee pot were also on the counter. This was all free. And it was very convenient—even the guests didn't need to go to the cafeteria. Again, it was nice, comfortable, and impressive. How thoughtful.

In addition, the nurses were attentive and came within minutes of my pressing the call bell. Each nurse was stationed in the hallway and was assigned to five rooms. This was a first for me. Usually, there is a nurse's station in the middle of the hall, with nurses who could never be found, or it would take them an hour to answer the call bell. I did not have to wait long here. The floor was quiet—there were no distracting noises, no alarms going off, no screaming, yelling, or "help me" noises coming from the rooms. This was so different from all my previous experiences.

Day three came, and it was discharge day. Time to go home.

I had a follow-up appointment for the following month to discuss the pathology report and options with the medical oncologist. Now, I had to heal again. Again, stay away from people, don't go out, don't let anyone come over, reduce all possible chance for infection. I had all this to worry about; plus, now I needed to adjust to having an uneven chest, with one implant and one side flat. How was I supposed to wear clothes? Could the flat side be repaired? How, and when? None of my shirts would fit me anymore. I went from a natural DD to barely an A on the left to nothing on the right. Scoop necks were out of the question, deep Vs were now too low cut. T-shirts looked horrible, as I could so easily notice the difference. A camisole or tank top needed a loose fit and a kimono over it to help distract. I learned how to fill the flat side with socks—I had to try to match the left side somehow. Some days, it was a one-sock day, others a two-sock ball, depending on what I wore.

How was I supposed to wear clothes? Would I do the chemo here, or where I lived? The doctor left it up to me. I asked to see the infusion suite, and I was in love. Now, this was how chemo should be: your own private room, with a TV, bed, and extra chair for a visitor. Also, you got a boxed lunch every day. Wow! I didn't have to sit around next to strangers looking at them getting chemo, I didn't have to talk to others, and there was privacy! I was impressed, but I told the doctor I would get treatment where I lived. Being on chemo and having to drive four hours home being sick would not be the best decision.

The Port

I would need to have a new port put in for the second round of chemo. The breast surgeon at the Tampa facility would order it. What is a port and why is it needed, you ask? A port is a small device that is placed under the skin with a catheter that feeds into a large vein and into the heart itself. It is used intravenously to feed medication into the bloodstream.[16] It can also be used to draw blood.

This would be an outpatient day surgery, scheduled on a Friday. I was all prepped and ready to go. Then I was asked: "Do you want to be sedated?" What type of question is that? Do you think I want to see, feel, and hear what you are doing? Do you think I would actually remain still while you come at me with a scalpel? Of course I want sedation!

The doctor told me the port would be on the left side of my chest, just under my collarbone. I was fine with that. I asked if they could use the same site that was used previously, and the answer was: "Sure, don't worry.

We will use the same scar line." Well, when I awoke, the port was under my right collarbone. What the heck! Why was it on my right side? It was supposed to be on the left. Again, mom was with me for this procedure as well. I started screaming and had the surgical team call the doctor for a removal order. This was not what I had consented to.

I found out that the reason it was put on the right side was that my veins were "torturous," and they couldn't get the port catheter in my veins, so they switched sides. I was livid—nothing like switching sides was ever mentioned. Who were they to take it upon themselves and switch sides? My mom was there—they could have asked her. She was on my paperwork and just in the waiting room. Did they? No! There was nothing but frustration, all the time, and always a complication. I guess the right side was it. The order did not give removal orders, so now I was stuck with a right-sided port and nothing more could be done. Home I went.

I knew recovery time was about a week. However, I didn't even make it that long. I started itching the very next day. The area of course was still sore and red. As was to be expected, the itching was uncontrollable. I took Benadryl, but it didn't help much. I thought I was allergic to the skin cleanser they'd used. So I waited until the next day to shower, as my paperwork specified no shower until day two. After I'd showered and thoroughly washed the area, the itch continued. So it wasn't the skin cleanser—was it the Steri-Strips I was allergic to? My skin and chest did show all the signs of an allergic reaction. So, I phoned the "on-call" number and spoke to the head of the Interventional Radiology (IR) Department. He sent me to my local emergency room for the possible allergic reaction, as today was Sunday. He also told me to call him back with the diagnosis. Okay, off to the ER I went.

The local ER saw me and treated me for the allergic reaction. I had the entire protocol for allergic reactions. The itch was still there. A chest rash, which spread to my waist and down my arm to the elbow, now also developed. The ER doctor thought I was allergic to the Steri-Strips, so those were removed. The medications that I was given didn't help with the symptoms. The conclusion: I was allergic to the port itself! Now, it had to come out. I called the IR doctor back and told him. He told me to return to Tampa the next day to have it taken out. So much for the right-sided port!

I was in preop going over the paperwork for the port removal with the nurses. I had a physician assistant (PA) who came to the bedside to say it would be about five minutes before I went back. "No problem," I said.

Three minutes later, a doctor came in and asked to see my problem area. I showed him and told him that they should be taking me back any minute. He stepped out from behind the curtain, talked to someone, and said, "No, you're not going back in a few minutes." What? Why not? He said: "I talked to you on the phone yesterday. I am ordering a bigger OR suite, and I will be taking out your port and putting another one in on the left side. The new one is a different material as well. I see about one case a year where people are allergic to the port." Of course, I had to be the one case.

Here we go again. My anxiety was going up. What about my "torturous veins"? I got another "don't worry" answer. I asked about sedation. You will get some, the doctor said. Good! The nurse started me with some "happy juice," but I still had high anxiety. How long before he could get a bigger OR suite? Would I really have a left-sided port? How did I know I could trust this doctor? What would happen if I was allergic to the new port? Would this happen again? It took about 20 minutes for the suite to be ready for me.

During this time, my anxiety was still very high. Once I was in the OR, the nurse told me she would give me sedation. I was waiting for it to kick in. The doctor explained everything to me, step by step. I saw, heard, and spoke to the doctor during the procedure. I felt pressure, but no pain. I was told to keep my head turned to the right. I kept wondering when the sedation would kick in? The doctor kept telling the nurse to give me more meds. I don't recall the dosage, what medications, or how much she gave me, but I do know that I was talking to the doctor during the entire procedure. I never went to sleep or felt relaxed.

When I got to the recovery room, mom was there waiting for me. She thought I would be groggy, but I told her I never went to "sleep." The doctor took out the right-sided port and got through my torturous veins on the left. The nurse proceeded to tell mom that she never saw anyone who fought sleep as much as I had. I had enough medication to keep me out for days.

We spent the night at a hotel after this ordeal. I took a four-hour nap. Sure, all the meds finally caught up to me. I was sore, groggy, and tired, but I managed. We had a four-hour drive home in the morning. Finally, the port issue was settled. Now that I had the port, it was time to start chemo. Of course, as with any port, there were some discomforts. Having a port on the left side does interfere with driving. The seat belt across the chest causes some pressure and soreness. I was fortunate to have a small port pillow attached to the seat belt. This allowed cushioning between the port and the belt.

Another port concern is discomfort, which occurs when the port is being accessed. It is an initial "sting," like when you're having a blood draw. The breakthrough of the skin is painful. Topical medications can be prescribed to help ease the sting. With this comes the potential for infection as well. Each time the port is accessed, the chances of infection increase. There is now a small opening in the skin, which can cause infection. Pain, redness, and swelling at the site are potential complications.

The Chemotherapy

I didn't want to go back to the oncologist I'd seen two years before, the "don't interrupt me" doctor, so I found a new group in my community. This new local doctor was nicer, allowed me to ask questions freely, still treated the cancer aggressively, and would follow all recommendations that the Tampa facility suggested. I would also need to find a local radiation doctor who would do the same, which I did. I wouldn't even need to worry about radiation until I finished another 16 weeks of chemo.

My new chemo plan was three days a week, every three weeks, for 16 cycles of dreaded chemo. Oh, how I hated going. To sit in the big room, with about 27 older and sick patients, who look like death warmed over, was not for me. I mean, if you are 97 years old, on oxygen, and have advanced-stage cancer, why would you opt for chemo? Why be chained to the doctor's office for three days a week? Who wants to experience all the nausea, hair loss, fatigue, and lab work—and for what? Was all this worth living an extra year or two? Not to me! I think these people should start looking at "buying a box" if they don't already have one. This was my way of saying they should have their caskets picked out and funeral arrangements made. Seriously, if the funeral homes would set up a table at the chemo office, I think sales would go up tremendously!Most of these people were older, sick people. After all, I live in Florida! I think many of them saw chemo as their "social club." Not me—I didn't want to talk to anyone. If mom or Elizabeth came, I would talk only to them. I don't think it was right that the entire room could hear your conversations. I wasn't there to make friends. I didn't want them knowing my story. I didn't want to compare notes, and I sure didn't even want to look at them. I tried to pick a chair out of the way, in a corner, and hide out. I didn't want to be looked at, either. I brought a coloring book and colored pencils to pass the usual four-hour session. This did the trick. I worked on coloring, and people didn't talk to me. If they tried, I politely stated that I was busy. This place didn't even have a communal TV. I also learned to carry my own personal blanket with me. This has its own separate story, which will be recounted shortly.

In retrospect, I knew why there was a blanket in the "goodie bag." It had to be a smart person who put it in there. First off, the facility was air-conditioned. It was on the cold side. Even with a sweater, it was cold. The blanket helped with comfort. Second, the chemo fluids were cold and lowered the body temperature. The blanket kept me warmer than I would have been without it. Third, the other option to help pass the time was to sleep. The blanket served its purpose here, too. As for me, I refused to sleep. I didn't trust the nurses. I wanted to ensure that all the medications were actually mine, so I had to watch to make sure there weren't any mistakes made. I had been through too much to not pay attention now. And yes, I fought off that Benadryl. It was a struggle, but I didn't sleep.

The Blanket

So back to the blanket story. The facility did have some spare blankets in the corner. I had seen them there on day one. I was chilly and eyed them, but I didn't say anything. Since I had a new blanket in my goodie bag, I used that one. I went home and washed my blanket, and then brought it again to the next visit. The reason I say a smart person put it in the bag was because of the circumstance of the blankets in the corner. The corner stack was quite large. The tower started on the floor and climbed up to the level of a chair railing. In my view, these blankets were dirty. Next, people were using them, and then putting them back on the pile. Hello! Anyone see any issue with this? Perhaps the rest of the pile is now "contaminated." How about this: Chemo patients are immunocompromised—what if germs spread? Those blankets were not laundered. They were used and put back. Duh, and gross! I refused to use those blankets. That is why I said that a smart person put the blanket in the goodie bag. They knew better. Smart people like me would use the one blanket during treatment, go home, wash it, and then bring it to the next appointment. It was dust-free, clean, and not touched by anyone but me.

My chemo treatment week took a toll. I would be sick with chemo during the chemo week and the following week. Just when I started to feel better, it was a chemo week. Mom stopped going with me after the first cycle, as this new place didn't allow her to stay with me. However, that was fine. Elizabeth, one of my good friends, volunteered to take me. She was so kind to pick me up, wait for with me during my four-hour treatment, and then treat me to lunch. She also sent me encouraging greeting cards in the interim as well. Elizabeth is extremely nice, thoughtful, supportive, and caring. I am so thankful to have her as a friend.

I had learned through my dad's cancer experience and my cancer experience two years before that—if I were terminal—I wanted quality of life over quantity of life. I wanted to be able to feel well, enjoy life, come and go, spend time with other people, and travel. Actually, with my health complications, cancer diagnosis, and surgeries, I seriously didn't think I would see age 45.

Once all the chemo treatments were completed, it was time to start radiation. September 2019 was the start of the 12-week radiation schedule. This was an everyday (Monday through Friday) schedule. This would be my first experience with radiation treatment. Previously, I didn't make it to the radiation stage before the recurrence happened. This was uncharted territory. I had to research radiation therapy to see what exactly I was in for. I heard many different views and expectations about it. The most common was that it was no big deal.

CHAPTER 3

Radiation: No Big Deal

The Basic Info

There are different variations and uses of radiation when it comes to cancer. First, what is radiation therapy?

Radiation therapy for breast cancer uses high-energy X-rays, protons, or other particles to kill cancer cells.[12] Delivery of radiation can be done in two ways: externally or internally.

External Radiation

External radiation is the most common type of radiation therapy used for breast cancer treatment. In this method, a machine delivers painless and invisible radiation from outside your body to the chest area and breast.

There are variations of external radiation therapy as well. A modified version is known as 3D conformal therapy. In this therapy, beams of radiation are created to match the shape of the tumor. This method allows for a decrease in exposure of healthy tissue and treats the tumor more accurately. With the increased precision, a higher dose of radiation can be used, and tumors can be destroyed more rapidly and effectively.

Intensity modulated radiation therapy (IMRT) is yet another advanced modification for external radiation. This technology manipulates the radiation beam and intensity of the radiation while conforming to the tumor's shape. This method helps to irradiate the tumor in a more accurate and precise manner. The goal here is similar to that of 3D conformal, where healthy tissue exposure and side effects are minimized.[13]

Internal Radiation (Brachytherapy)

Internal radiation, or brachytherapy, is a treatment in which radiation seeds or pellets are inserted within the body at the tumor site. These seeds or pellets are temporary. The radiation source is then placed over the seeds or pellets during the treatment. Once the course of treatment is complete, the seeds or pellets can be surgically removed.

No matter what method is used, radiation therapy may be used at any stage of breast cancer. It can be used prior to surgery, after surgery, and sometimes instead of surgery. Radiation therapy is usually used after surgery to help reduce the risk of the breast cancer returning. In addition, radiation therapy can also be used to help ease the symptoms caused by cancer that has spread to other parts of the body (metastatic breast cancer).[12] Why is this? Simply put, radiation therapy kills cancer cells.

Photon radiation is another type of radiation treatment that is being researched for the management and treatment of patients with early-stage and locally advanced breast cancer. My research concluded that photon radiation has not been shown to be any more effective than traditional radiation treatments, and can cost 4 to 10 more than traditional radiation. However, photon radiation for breast cancer is still under investigation. My focus will be on external radiation with IMRT for mastectomy and locally advanced breast cancer, as this was my experience.

Radiation After Mastectomy

Radiation may also be used after mastectomy. Just because the entire breast has been removed with a mastectomy, this does not eliminate the risk of recurrence. Recurrence can occur in any remaining tissue of the chest wall or surrounding lymph nodes.

In many situations, the risk of recurrence is high, and radiation after mastectomy is highly recommended. This type of radiation is called post-mastectomy radiation therapy. The therapy is typically administered on a daily basis for about 6 to 12 weeks.

One factor that indicates a higher risk of breast cancer recurrence includes the chest wall or lymph nodes testing positive during biopsy or during surgery. If so, there is a higher indication for radiation after mastectomy. Radiation therapy may also be suggested when:

- The underarm (axillary) lymph nodes test positive for cancer. This can be a sign that some cancer cells have spread from the primary tumor.[12]

- The tumor size is large, meaning greater than about 2 inches (5 centimeters). This carries a significantly higher risk for recurrence than smaller tumors do.[12]

- Positive tissue margins also aid in the suggestion for radiation therapy. When breast tissue is removed, it is examined by a pathologist, and its margins are also examined for any remaining signs of cancer cells. If the pathology determines very narrow margins or positive margins, there is a higher risk for recurrence, and radiation therapy is strongly suggested.[12]

Radiation for Inflammatory Breast Cancer

Radiation can also be used to treat advanced breast cancer. The intent of the radiation treatment is to reduce the size of breast tumors. Inflammatory breast cancer can also benefit from radiation therapy. Inflammatory breast cancer is an aggressive type of breast cancer that spreads through the skin and to the to the lymph channels of the breast. The typical recommended treatment plan for people with inflammatory breast cancer is chemotherapy prior to having a mastectomy, followed by radiation therapy to decrease the chance of recurrence.[12] My grandmother had inflammatory breast cancer.

Radiation for Managing Metastatic Breast Cancer

Radiation can also be used to manage metastatic breast cancer. Breast cancer is metastatic if it has *metastasized*—spread from the point of origin to other parts of the body. Pain can occur, and radiation therapy can be used to shrink the tumor and ease those symptoms.[12]

My experience with radiation after a double mastectomy is somewhat limited. Why, you ask? It is because I decided at the last minute (after a form was created and I had radiation tattoos on me) that I was not going to pursue radiation therapy. I had many reasons for this. One reason was that a year had passed before radiation would start. Why start now? If I didn't have cancer or a recurrence, why was radiation so important? Why would I want to start radiation after a year of being cancer free?

Second, I was in "remission." And third, I had a radiation oncologist whom I didn't trust. How could I be sure he knew what he was doing, when he couldn't answer my questions about radiation therapy? My questions were similar to those I asked of the medical oncologist:

"What is the percentage chance that this treatment would be effective?"

"What are my chances that breast cancer will return?"

"How many sessions will I need to attend?"

"Umm, let's see what happens and play it out," was not an answer that gave me confidence. Dumbass doctor! Also, he proceeded to tell me that he needed to go and look up the percentage in a book in the other room.

"Fine, go," I told him. "I'll wait."

After about a five-minute break, he came back in with some small book and turned to some random page and said: "Well, it states that for your age and type of cancer, your percentage is 50 percent."

So I asked: "Can I see the book and the graph?"

He said "no," closed the book, and walked out of the room. Mom and I just looked at each other and asked: "Is he coming back?"

The answer was a clear "no." We waited for about another five minutes in the office, wondering if he would return, but he never did. That was the end of that doctor. If the chance was 50 percent, then why wouldn't I take the chance and not have the radiation done, with the hope that I had half a chance the cancer would not recur?

Now, three years later, unfortunately, my cancer did recur, and having been diagnosed with locally advanced breast cancer, I have experience with radiation therapy and am faced with daily radiation treatments. It is either do this or risk having a third recurrence. Twice is enough—I don't want to experience breast cancer a third time. I now have a new radiation oncologist who provided competent answers to my questions and concerns.

I did ask the question: "What if I don't do radiation therapy?"

The answer was, "If you don't, your chances are 99.9 percent recurrence in the next six months."

My follow-up question was: "What is my percentage it will not return if I do radiation?" This was a fair enough question, I thought. The answer was not so straightforward.

"Well, I can't give you a percentage. However, it is much lower than not doing it—maybe cut in a third." So, if I was 99 percent without radiation, now it was down to 33 percent? I guessed that was better odds than having cancer back in six months. Option one was take the radiation and decrease the risk. Option two was do nothing and get cancer for a possible third time. I decided to take option one and have the radiation. I hope that after all this, I will be in the 66 percent of patients in whom radiation killed all the cancerous cells, and I will be cancer-free for many years to come.

Radiation therapy is not without side effects. So be sure you are not told"
"Radiation is no big deal—there is nothing to worry about."

If you are told this, Google it, say, "Let me think about it," and leave
the office. Radiation has side effects. This is one of the reasons why, as
mentioned earlier, I did not want radiation to begin with. Side effects for
radiation include: constant tiredness, skin irritation, and chronic fatigue.[14]
The constant tiredness and fatigue are daily occurrences, and afternoon
naps are a must. The chest wall and breast skin in the treatment areas become dry, red, discolored, more sensitive, and in some cases even swollen.
Other skin changes can include dryness. There is a constant need to apply
lotions, creams, and ointments. Itching, peeling, blistering, and other skin
issues can occur as well. But again, lotions, creams, and ointments may be
recommended for use.

Depending on the area being treated, other early side effects may include:

- Loss of hair in or around the treatment area.

- Dry mouth, which can lead to a difficulty in swallowing.

- Lack of appetite.

- Digestive problems, such as nausea, vomiting, and diarrhea.

- Increase in headaches or migraines.

- Tenderness, redness, and swelling in the treatment area.

- Increase or decrease in urinary output.

Late side effects, which are rare, occur months or years following treatment.
They are more often permanent in nature. They can include changes to the:

- Brain

- Spinal cord

- Lungs

- Kidneys

- Colon

- Joints[3]

Long-term effects can also include:

- Lymphedema—swelling in the arm and hand

- Infertility

- Secondary cancer[3]

Keep in mind that radiation therapy can also cause a slight chance of a secondary cancer from the radiation itself. Regular follow-up visits with the radiation oncologist can help prevent any of these complications from occurring. Using advanced technologies, such as IMRT, radiation oncologists can help maximize the cancer-destroying capabilities of radiation treatment while minimizing its effects on healthy tissues and organs.

Preparation for Radiation

The first step is simulation. This is where you are "casted and marked" for daily therapy. You are asked to lie on the computed axial tomography (CAT) scan table with a foam pillow and positioned for the target area to be marked. During this process, once you're positioned, the foam pillow is molded to your body. It will be used daily for perfect positioning. Also, small lead wires are taped to your chest, and a CAT scan is obtained to plan treatment for the target area. After the CAT scan, the taped lead wires are removed, and small permanent radiation tattoos are placed on your body. These tattoos are done with a lancet and some food dye. (I had three on my torso.) These tattoos also serve as position markers for daily radiation delivery. The only part the patient feels is the permanent tattooing process. From here, the CAT scan images are reviewed by the radiation oncologist, who establishes the treatment plan. This process usually takes about two weeks. Then the first treatment will start.

The Schedule

The first two weeks are like nothing. This is when the expression "radiation is no big deal" comes into play. After that, however, the side effects of radiation start to occur. Skin darkening, loss of hair, fatigue, and soreness in the treatment were what I experienced. Every day—and by "every day" I mean Monday through Friday—my treated area hurt more and more. Rib and chest wall soreness got so bad, I couldn't touch the treatment area. The slightest pressure made me jump off the exam table. The pressure of a shirt was too much, but I had to wear one—I couldn't walk around topless! Every day I went for treatment for what was supposed to be eight weeks. Notice I wrote "supposed "to be." Has any part of this story been straightforward and simple? Of course not.

The first two weeks were fine. At the start of week three there was a hurricane, so that was four days off, through no fault of my own. That just added four additional days at the end of the eight weeks—make-up days. I started back for the third week, and the radiation exam room door broke. The door didn't close, and there was no radiation treatment for another two days—the door had to be fixed. That added two more make-up days to the supposed end date.

During week four, I started to blister and get radiation burns. I was told I had shingles. So now that I was contagious with shingles, I needed to take 10 days off. I didn't believe I had shingles—I thought it was just radiation blisters and burns. But I followed the shingles protocol.

I had antibiotics, no radiation, and quarantine for 10 days, adding another 10 make-up days. Finally, I got back to radiation with more crusted-over "shingles pox," and after two more days of radiation the "shingles" were back and with a vengeance. Now, the "shingles" were more prevalent, and oozing. I still though they were radiation burns, but I was told it wasn't burned—it was a second bout of shingles. Why would my condition get worse with the radiation treatment? Why wouldn't the radiation help dry up the shingles?

Hmm. If it was radiation burns, it only made sense that more radiation would worsen the condition, doesn't it? Here is a photo—you decide. Radiation burn or shingles?

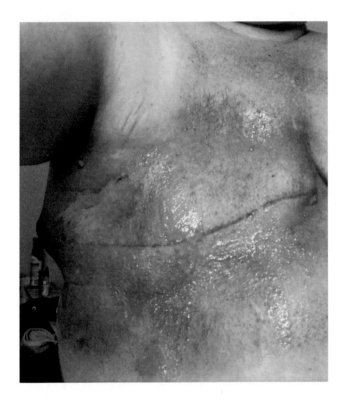

Again, I was told it was shingles. Oh, great! A second course of antibiotics, no radiation for a week, and quarantine again—more make-up days for me. When would I get done with radiation? Was there a radiation end date in sight? Not that I could see.

CHAPTER 4

The Hospital Visit

just saw the doctor the previous day in the office. On October 20, 2019, I went in for my daily radiation treatment but didn't feel well. I had some oozing from my chest. I saw the doctor, who told me I was in the "wet stage," and that was normal. He offered me the day off from radiation, and I took it. I didn't feel well. I went home, carried on the day normally, ran a few errands, tended to the dog, and went to bed.

I woke up on the morning of October 22, 2019 cold as could be. I took a shower, which didn't help me to get warm. I felt nauseous and saw a purplish rash on my stomach. Oh great—something new. After brushing my teeth, I got dressed, then threw up. Something was wrong. I was sick, cold with chills, shakes, a new purple rash, and vomiting. I got dressed and drove myself to the doctor's office. Since I had to have blood work, what better place to be? Well, I ended up throwing up outside the office door where the nurses came to get me in a wheelchair and took me in.

They took my temperature and told me it was 101. I was to go to the emergency room. I never saw the doctor, just a nurse who wheeled me back to my car. I drove back across town with a puke bag in one hand and threw up at traffic lights. Fifteen minutes later, I got to the free-standing ER near my house. I walked in and said I was a cancer patient who was sick. I was triaged right away—no need to fill out paperwork right now. I handed over my green bile vomit, and they took my temperature (101.5 degrees), blood pressure (150/96), and pulse (104). Straight back to the ER bay I went. The nurse and doctor came right in. I told them my symptoms, and showed them my oozing "shingles" and the new purple rash.

The ER doctor said: "You are getting admitted now!" This ER physician told me I had severe radiation burns. Finally! It was only about 11:30 a.m. The medical team was on top of me; they took my blood, asked for urine, cultured my oozing and seeping radiation burns, and sent me for a CT of the abdomen. I wasn't even sure what was wrong with me. The doctor told me I had bad radiation burns with cellulitis. I was in severe sepsis.

Oh my God! That was bad. I was extremely sick. They told me they would transfer me to the hospital in a few hours. Well, those turned out to be a long few hours. It was 8 p.m. before the ambulance came for me. Mind you, I had arrived at the ER at 11:30 a.m.! Sorry, but that is more than just a "few hours."

Finally, transport came for me. The paramedic introduced himself and said: "I remember you—you were my teacher in EMT school. You made me do 80 push-ups." Oh boy! That was three years before.

I said: "Well, at least I know you were trained well." He did take good care of me and kept me informed. Overall, it was a good, short transport experience. You never know who you may meet when or what your legacy may be.

Anyway, I got into the hospital bed in my private isolation room, and I was out. I was so sick those first three days in the hospital that I hardly remember them. All I remember is the nurses coming in and taking my temperature, followed by Tylenol. Every time they came in, my fever was going higher and higher. I remember 103.4 degrees but was later told the highest was 104! Along with this, I did not get to sleep soundly at night either. I woke up in pain—my chest and ribs were so sore that I couldn't lie on them. I was also awakened for blood draws.

"Code blue" (life-threatening medical emergency, such as cardiac or respiratory arrest) and "code gray" (request for hospital security personnel) announcements were other nightly disturbances. Call bells were going off in the hallway all night as well. The nurses were hardly around and did not respond quickly to those call bells at all. Since when is it that if you don't ask for pain medicine, you don't get any? In all my prior pain experiences in the hospital, a patient would get pain medicine every four to six hours, needed or not. I knew there was an opioid epidemic, but hello, I was in the hospital. Isn't it the nurse's job to administer medications, monitor the patient's pain levels, record medication times, and document any reactions?

Let's not even get me started on the nurses. Where were they all night? I thought they had a secret hideout room. They were never around. It took more than 30 minutes for them to answer a call bell. Did they actually have experience? Many of them were fresh out of nursing school, with less than a year of experience. They looked so young. Did they have the necessary knowledge to care for me? This was not only the nurses, but also the patient care techs (PCTs), the people who bring you water and draw blood.

Another bad experience was blood draws at the bedside. Since the surgery, my right arm was off-limits for blood draws due to lymphedema. For three days and nights, a PCT would come in to draw my blood. She would reach for my right arm as the left was attached to the blood pressure machine. I would say, "*No*. You can't use that arm; it has to be the left arm."

She said "Okay," and went to the left arm for the specimen. Day in and day out for three days, it was the same conversation with many PCTs. Did any of them ask why no right arm? *No*. Did any of them say ask, "Where is your 'restricted arm' band?" No. Did any of them report it to the nurse? No. It was not until day four, when I went to preop for port removal, that the nurses said: "You don't have a band?"

My answer was *No*. I had been telling them on the floor for three days, and nothing. Good thing the OR nurse banded me.

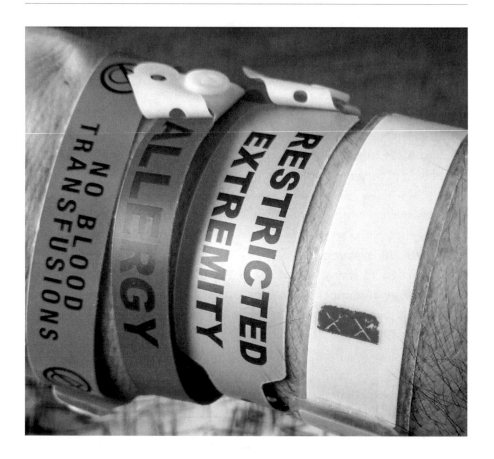

Finally, smart nurses!

After the third night, I learned that it was better to stay up in the middle of the night and sleep in the morning, starting at 7 a.m. after shift change until noon, and then again from 2 to 6 p.m. These hours offered the best option for sleep, but still not the greatest. I think it was days four and five that I was actually sleeping from 7 to 11 a.m. Even with that, I was awakened to see if I wanted to order breakfast. The answer was "*No.*" I heard my room phone ring, but ignored it. Since I didn't answer the phone, the breakfast department called the nurses' station. The nurse had to wake me up to see if I was skipping breakfast. Did they think I was dead because I didn't answer the phone? Really, come on. Dumb. Then around 9 o'clock, I was awakened again when the doctor finally came in for rounds. Once I started to fall asleep again, there came the knock on the door for the cleaning person.

Did you think I was going to sleep when there was a cleaning person in the room? *No!* I had to watch them to ensure that they didn't steal from me. I would sleep shortly after they left. All in all, it was a terrible sleep experience in the hospital. I followed this routine for seven nights. On day eight, I finally felt "better" and asked about my discharge. At this point, I was on IV antibiotics for 30 minutes twice a day. Why did I still need to be here? Why couldn't I go home?

I was told this was because I needed another 10 days of antibiotics. So I was supposed to stay in the hospital for another 10 days just to get this antibiotic for 30 minutes twice a day? The answer was "Yes."

"Heck, no!" I replied. I would rather be at home with my own germs than in here. Shortly after that, the discharge planner was called in to discuss my discharge. He stated that he could set up home care, but if I wanted to speed up the process I could call and try to set it up as well. On the phone I went. Two wasted hours got me nowhere. Why was I doing this from my bed? What else did I have to do? What was the discharge planner's job? So, needless to say, I spent another night in the hospital because nothing was accomplished. The next morning, the discharge planner came in about 9 a.m. and said I was going home today at about 11 a.m. Great! I got dressed, called for a ride, and then came to find out it would be another four hours until I could actually leave.

I ordered lunch and waited for the time to pass. The discharge guy came in about 4 p.m. and said everything was set up and I could go home. I pressed the call button for the nurse. No answer. Finally, about 30 minutes later the nurse came in and asked what I needed. "Discharge papers," I said.

"Oh, you're going home today?" she asked.

"Yes!" I replied.

"Okay," she said. "Let me work on the papers." Another hour later, she came in and had me sign everything. She told me to wait for the wheel-chair, which should be here shortly. I was waiting, waiting, and waiting—no wheelchair. Mom went to look for a nurse—of course, no nurses were in sight—I guess they are hiding out again. I pressed the call button. A PCT came in, and I said I needed a wheelchair to go home. She said she would call for transport. Waiting, waiting, and waiting some more. It was another hour before the wheelchair came. Now it was 8 p.m. at discharge time. I had been ready since 11 a.m., and I couldn't wait to get home.

The Home Nurses

Finally, I made it home after 10 days in the hospital. Ah! My own bed, and a bed at that, not a 2-inch-thick mattress that I had been "sleeping" on for 10 days. Well, as much as I wanted the bed, I retreated to the recliner couch instead. With a midline IV in my arm for the at-home antibiotics and a right chest that was still very painful, the couch was more comfort-able. I slept from 9 p.m. that night until 8 a.m. the next morning. Finally, a quiet and restful night.

I had to wake up early for the FedEx shipment of IV supplies and medi-cations. If I didn't sign, it would have gone back. Delivery was scheduled between 8 a.m. and 11 a.m. From there, the visiting nurse was to come over from noon to 2 p.m. She would show me how to set up, administer, and take care of the midline. This midline was no joke. It is similar to an IV in your hand, but it is in the bend of my elbow. The end was taped up, so I could reach it. It was wrapped in cling with supportive cotton braces holding it all in place. Then it had a mesh sleeve on the top to keep it clean. Of course, I am allergic to tapes and adhesive, so these creative, abstract, makeshift coverings were not standard practice.

The visiting nurse came and went through all the FedEx materials with me. She showed me how to clean the IV port, administer the medications, and evaluate the site for any potential issues. I told her I knew how to do this. I was a healthcare provider: a paramedic, certified medical assistant, x-ray tech, and a pharm tech. Besides, I taught these subjects. With that, she seemed comfortable with coming to visit me every few days rather than every day. I had to administer the IV twice a day for 10 days. She returned two days later—October 31, 2019 to be exact—to change the dressing on the IV. Again, creativity was needed. Tape and adhesive could not touch my skin. My arm was sore and felt uncomfortable for the rest of the afternoon.

After dinner, the trick-or-treaters started ringing the bell. I had this monstrous wrapped IV protruding from my arm. Everyone thought it was a great "costume." It was no costume, it was the real thing! Around 8 p.m., the trick-or-treaters were still going strong. My candy bowl was getting low. I went to refill the candy bowl and noticed the IV catheter was starting to come out of my arm. Oh, no! This was not good. I grabbed a saline flush, sat down, and tried to flush the IV. It would not flush. I tried "floating" the IV in—still no good. The IV started bleeding at the site. Quickly, I phoned the nurses on call and told them I had three more days of medications to go, and my IV was coming out. They told me to go to the ER.

How was I supposed to get there? My entire arm was bandaged from shoulder to wrist. I had to apply pressure to the elbow to stop the bleeding from the IV. Who should I call? I called mom, who lived only five minutes from me.

I asked: "Can you take me to the ER?"

"When?" she replied.

"Now!" I said.

"Now? You want me to take you now? At 8 p.m. on Halloween night? With trick-or-treaters on the streets?"

Uh, yes. Why would I call now, if I wanted you to take me tomorrow? I needed to go now. The IV was coming out of my arm and bleeding.

Mom said, "Okay, I will be right over." Who plans on going to the ER a day before they want to go? I thought it was funny. But from mom's perspective, I can see how she needed to stop what she was doing, get in the car, and drive over.

The Emergency Room (ER)

To the ER I went, on Halloween night. Don't worry, I did bring some "treat bags" for the nurses and staff. Again, I was able to go right in. I didn't need to fill out any paperwork, as I had an IV bleeding from my arm. They took my vitals and brought me to the exam room. The doctor came in and recognized me from the previous week when I had gone in with sepsis. I told her the IV was coming out. I was trying to save it, tried to float it in, but to no avail. I think it just needed to be removed and replaced. The emergency room doctor examined the IV, consulted with the nurse, and then asked me how many more doses of antibiotics I had left to take. I told her I had three more days to go. They concluded the best way to handle this situation was to take out the midline. That is what I thought would happen, but I needed it legally documented. This way, it didn't look as though I pulled it out myself or was noncompliant. It was now on record that I had the midline in place with a complication when I walked into the ER.

Here is the kicker: They could not replace this midline with a new one. They took it out, but told me I needed to go to a different hospital, and through the ER, to get another one put in. Hello, it was now 10 p.m. on Halloween night. Plus the other hospital was owned by the same company. What kind of hospital says "We don't have the ability to place a midline here?" This one. Did they think I was willing to travel 20 minutes across town at 10 p.m. on Halloween night to go and get a new one? Seriously! No way. My arm was just starting to feel relief from not having the midline in. The bulking bandage was off. I had mobility of my full arm. This was great. Arm freedom! Would three more days of antibiotics make that much of a difference? The answer was no. Mom drove me home after the midline removal, and I went to bed with a freed arm.

The next day, I wondered. Hmm, should I go and spend the next several hours in an ER waiting for a midline, or forget it? I phoned the on-call nurses and told them what had happened the previous night. I canceled the day's visit. There was no reason for them to come if I didn't need to be evaluated. I decided not to go to the ER for another midline, not to continue the last three days of medications, and not to have the home nurse come anymore.

I felt fine. My body had been through enough. I didn't want to look or feel sick anymore. I just wanted to be left alone. I was tired of all the tests, poking, prodding, and fuss. If I was going to die, I wanted to die without all this going on. However, I felt that I was on the mend. I was home, my burns were starting to heal up, and I had some energy—all steps in the road to recovery.

The Follow-ups

The next few weeks were booked with follow-up appointments with various doctors: one with the infectious diseases (ID) doctor, one with primary care, one with the medical oncologist, and another radiation oncologist. The ID doctor was a joke. I saw this doctor twice in the hospital, and now I had to go to her office to double-check that I was well. I did mention about not finishing the last three days of antibiotic because of the midline complications. She said that since I was on it longer than seven days and felt well, all was well. Hooray! No need to go back to that office again. As it was, that office was located on the second floor of a medical building. The office wallpaper was peeling. The other patients looked sick. Many of them looked like stereotypical, classic AIDS/HIV patients. They looked thin and malnourished. This was a scary place, and one I didn't want to return to.

The appointment with the primary care physician was a good one. She was concerned about my health, my well-being, and my hospital test results. She also wanted to coordinate care with the medical oncologist and radiation oncologist. She gave me good advice about trying to gain more weight and my malnutrition status. I'd lost more than 15 pounds in the hospital over the 10 days I was there. The weight loss was too rapid, and I became malnourished. I just didn't feel like eating, and who enjoys hospital food? During the upcoming holidays, I was told to "indulge" to help get my weight stabilized. The doctor also ordered additional lab work to ensure that my body was recovering. Lab results would dictate the next appointment. As for now, she scheduled me for a three-month follow-up.

The follow-up with the medical oncologist was okay. Now that surgery was completed and chemo and radiation were over with, it was time to start hormone blocker, tamoxifen. Tamoxifen is in the selective estrogen receptor modulator (SERM) class of medications. It is a hormonal therapy.[17] SERMs work by blocking the effects of estrogen in the breast tissue by attaching to the estrogen receptors in breast cells. Tamoxifen is a popular medication in this class, used to treat men and both premenopausal and postmenopausal women. It is typically used to:

- Reduce the risk of recurrence in early-stage breast cancer with positive hormone receptors from coming back after surgery and other treatments.

- Aid in the shrinkage of tumors prior to surgery.

- Treat positive hormone receptor breast cancer.

- Reduce risk in undiagnosed women who are at higher-than-average risk of developing breast cancer.

Depending on a woman's menopausal status, tamoxifen is a 5- to 10-year hormonal treatment.[17] It was recommended that I go on this medication for 10 years. Here it was, now December 2019, just before Christmas, and I was to start this oral and daily medication. Off to the pharmacy I went.

The tamoxifen was a small pill that was easy to swallow, but after three days on it, the side effects started. Nausea, hot flashes, rapid heartbeat, and headache were the only side effects I experienced. How to combat these side effects? Would they dissipate in a few more days? Should I stop taking it? Should I take additional medications to suppress the side effects? Should I call the doctor? These were all valid questions that I considered. I decided to go with the drugs to treat the side effects. I had anti-nausea medicine and migraine medicine and took it for the following three days. No help.

I felt as though I didn't want to waste these medications on the side effects of the tamoxifen. What if I needed them for a real migraine? I couldn't take these medications every day, either. There are drawbacks as well, such as "rebound side effects." I could have additional headaches from taking headache medicine. How was I supposed to know then if it was a "real migraine/headache" or a "rebound migraine/headache"? I stopped the anti-nausea and migraine medications and just took the once-a-day tamoxifen. It had been 10 days. Side effects were still present, and additional ones started.

Now, my heart would race so hard that I would wake up from sleep. It was running so fast that it caused me to worry. Just what I needed—more stress—stress on top of stress. In addition, hot flashes would also wake me up. I'd get so sweaty that I would need to change my pajamas. The house temperature was set at 68 degrees Fahrenheit. This was cool, especially for living in Florida in the winter. Previously, I had the house thermometer set to 74 degrees to be comfortable. The hot flashes also occurred several times during the day, but the nights seemed to be worse. The nights were bad for the racing heart issue, too.

During the middle of the night, I would wake up with palpitations. My heart felt as though it would jump out of my chest. This is where my medical background came in handy. I tried to lie still and take my pulse. I wanted to assess the regularity and the number of beats per minute. I knew from my paramedic training that a new onset of atrial fibrillation (irregular heartbeat); sinus tachycardia (fast heart rate); paroxysmal supraventricular tachycardia (PSVT)—very fast heart rate; or ventricular tachycardia (abnormally fast heart rate in the lower portion of the heart) could potentially be deadly rhythms. I narrowed my possibilities down to sinus tachycardia or PSVT. This was based on the "regularity and heart rate" of my self-assessment. I tried what I know for treatment options: slow breathing, relaxation, and vagal maneuvers.

What are vagal maneuvers? A vagal maneuver is an action used to slow down the heart rate by stimulating the vagus nerve. The vagus nerve is part of the autonomic nervous system, which helps regulate many of the body's critical functions.[10] These functions include regulation of heart rate, blood pressure, sweating, and digestion.[10] When the vagus nerve is stimulated, it releases acetylcholine, which slows the pulse.[10] Simple procedures that can be performed to create a vagal response include holding one's breath, coughing, blowing through a straw, bearing down, and having cold water applied to the face.[18] For me, coughing worked the best. I felt my heart rhythm convert back to normal. Usually, if this didn't work, the next step would be medication control. After a month with all these symptoms, I reported them to my medical oncologist.

As I expected, I was referred to a cardiologist to check my heart for this new-onset arrhythmia. I was assigned to an Indian cardiologist who saw me for five minutes and ordered lab work, an echocardiogram (EKG), and a Holter monitor. My labs were all normal, including my electrolyte levels. (Low or high electrolytes can cause heart issues, too.) My EKG was normal, and the Holter monitor only showed sinus tachycardia (fast heart rate). The Holter monitor was a small, continuous EKG machine with electrodes attached to my chest. I wore this small device for 24 hours.

The follow-up with the cardiologist was another five-minute visit. "You are fine, nothing to do," he said. "If you get short of breath, or you feel worse, go to the ER." No kidding! Did he think I was going to wait on a situation like this? I know this is a serious issue, and I may need to be "converted." His advice was "get an Apple watch" to monitor your heart rate. "You can take an EKG when it acts up, upload it to me, and then go to the ER anyway."

No, thanks. I didn't want to wear a watch all the time, didn't want to spend more than $500 on the watch, and didn't want to do all the work the ER should have been doing. If I had a heart problem that didn't resolve itself within a few minutes, I'd go to the ER. Other than that, no meds. The doctor said the side effects would outweigh the benefits, so no cardiac meds for me.

I saw the medical oncologist again in January 2020. I reported to her the cardiology situation, and explained that the sinus tachycardia was still occurring. I mentioned the other side effects as well. She took me off the tamoxifen and put me on another hormone blocker called anastrozole, brand name Arimidex. When I explained my side effects, the doctor said she was not surprised that I had failed on Tamoxifen. Well, if she knew this would happen, why did she make me start it? Why waste a month? Why let me suffer with the side effects? Perhaps for another office visit? For another copay? To ensure I would report back that I had side effects? To document my failure to go to the next drug? For insurance to cover the next option?

Now it was on to anastrozole, aka Arimidex, which is used for postmenopausal women who have tested positive for hormones associated with locally advanced or metastatic breast cancers.[19] Arimidex is usually the first-line medication given to patients. It can also be used as a second-line treatment following the failure of Tamoxifen therapy.[19] There was yet another problem with me starting this medication—the key point being postmenopausal. I was not there yet. So already a problem, and I hadn't even started taking it yet. Lab tests were ordered to confirm that I was not yet menopausal. So, how would I get there? Goserelin acetate, sold under the brand name Zoladex, was how! Zoladex is another medication that can be used in the treatment of breast cancer for pre- and perimenopausal women.[19] This pellet looked like rabbit food and was given to me by injection just under the skin in my abdomen. The injection hurt, and a bruise followed for five days. This was needed to put me into menopause, so that the hormone blocker pill could work most efficiently. For one month, I just accepted the injection to reduce any potential side effects. The only thing I experienced was hot flashes. The following month, and not long after I started the Arimidex, additional side effects occurred.

The insomnia, hot flashes, confusion, headaches, and tachycardia continued. The insomnia was pretty bad. I would be up all day and all night. I would try to go to bed around 10 p.m. but tossed and turned. What was I to do? Well, I got up and tried to get tired. I did laundry, bleached kitchen counters, and then wrote some of this book. (How do you think this chapter was completed?) I would sometime stay up until 3 or 4 a.m. I would then start my day at 6 or 7 a.m. I knew my body needed sleep. It had not yet fully recovered from all this trauma. My immunity was still low, and now the insomnia was causing me headaches and confusion. Of course, this is what happens when your body needs sleep. I took this medicine until I saw the doctor again a month later. I thought that perhaps after a few weeks these side effect would subside. That was not that case. Actually, I think they got worse.

I went back to the doctors for the monthly injection and to report these side effects. Maybe I should not do anything. I'd rather not have debilitating side effects and feel good. From my research, I found that these hormone blockers reduce the cancer recurrence rate by only 30 percent. Was a 30 percent reduction enough? I thought the odds were in my favor. After all, this was already my second time. I'd been through enough. I'd had enough. I decided that, in the case of recurrence, I would not do anything about it anyway—just comfort measures—no more surgeries, no more chemo, no more radiation, nothing. Heck, I even completed and filed a do not resuscitate (DNR) order with my primary physician and medical oncologist. I was willing to chance it.

Of course, this did not go over so well with the doctor. However, she seemed to be understanding and had to do her due diligence. She told me that if I did not take a hormone blocker, I would be at high risk for recurrence. I knew that. I explained that I did not think the 30 percent reduction was high enough for me. I also told her my thoughts if it should come back. Her suggestion was that I try another medication, see how I do, and then decide. Although I had already make up my mind, I said okay. The third hormone blocker medication was letrozole.

Letrozole, sold as brand name Femara, is another medication used in the treatment of breast cancer. Letrozole is a nonsteroidal medication used for postmenopausal women works by lowering estrogen levels. Of course, the postmenopausal issue occurs again. I still needed to have the Zoladex injections into my abdomen every month. There seemed to be no chance of decreasing any medication anytime soon. Still, I had another month with new side effects from letrozole as well: night sweats, headaches, and nausea. Again, my thought process was the same as previously—maybe in a few weeks everything would settle down, and I would get use to this medication. Nope. The side effects continued. This was the third medication combination that I did not tolerate. Third times a charm for me.

That was it—I'd had enough! No more meds. I was tired of all the side effects from these medications. To suffer with them for the next 5 to 10 years was not going to happen. This was how long I would need to take them before I could discontinue them and be "cleared." This was way too much craziness for me, especially for only a 30 percent reduction. I'd been dealing with medication issues for the past three months. Enough!

It was March 2020. I took myself off all cancer medications. No nothing. Finally, I had some good luck. My medication side effects subsided. The hot flashes went away, and I had no more night sweats, insomnia, or confusion. The headaches decreased (just the occasional migraine), the nausea dissipated, and I started to feel "good." I still had some episodes of tachycardia, but that seemed to be improving as well. These were all good signs. Heck, I even thought I was now in natural menopause! I couldn't ask for better, right?

But my luck was short-lived and ran out. Coronavirus (COVID-19) hit the world. Everyone was on "safer at home" orders. Just when I thought I could go out and enjoy life, I couldn't. I hadn't been around a group of people in months—maybe even years—due to my poor immune system being constantly compromised. Now, there was a government restriction requiring people to stay home, and all social activities were canceled.

April 2020. I had my first video appointment with the medical oncologist—telemedicine at its finest due to COVID-19. Even the doctors' offices were closed, all elective surgeries were canceled, there were no face-to-face appointments, and 6 feet apart was the new personal space. It had been a month of COVID-19 already, and telemedicine was becoming the new standard. Anyway, my video appointment with the medical oncologist went better than expected. She asked how I felt, and my reply was "good."

I told her that most of the medication side effects eased up when I stopped taking them. She asked if I wanted to go back and try Tamoxifen again. I said "No." Why would I want to do that when I knew what the side effects were? That seemed to be a dumb question to ask me. She told me she respected my decision but did warn me that if the cancer returned, it would be my responsibility. Yes, I knew that, for the umpteenth time! I asked what would be next. Her reply was blood work and appointments every-three-months to help ensure my health. At this point, I was considered to be in "remission" and medically cleared to go back to work—but only part time. I was not cured, and not cancer-free. These terms are used only after five years of no additional cancer problems. I'll take remission!

I asked: "Am I still considered immunocompromised?"

She told me "no." However, she said I should follow the "safer at home" orders and wear a mask if I should go to the grocery store or pharmacy. Hmm, did that make sense? If I was not immunocompromised, why would I need to take such strict precautions? My labs showed I had a low white count (meaning I was immunocompromised, from what I know).

I told my brother that the doctor said I was not immunocompromised. He said: "Don't you know that doctors don't know diddly?" He went on to say, "Of course you are immunocompromised. You're a cancer patient, and you have a low white count." I loved it—now even my brother thought doctors made dumbass comments!

CHAPTER 5

Support From Family and Friends

Mom

I have to say that without the support of my family and friends I would not have been as strong as I was. My mom was there for me every step of the way. Mom started her own battle with breast cancer at the young age of 40, then lung cancer at the age of 61. Her breast cancer experience was similar to mine, and she too had a recurrence. She opted for lumpectomy, as her cancer was not invasive, unlike mine. She did the five years of tamoxifen, which didn't work. She had a recurrence as well. She opted for a second lumpectomy and stereotactic radiation therapy, with few side effects.

The lung cancer was caused by my dad's secondhand smoke and was very aggressive as well. She had to have an entire lung removed. Yes, you can live with one lung! She has had a clean bill of health for the past 10 years. Mom is a spunky, strong woman who is about to turn 71. She has much energy and is constantly on the go. She has been there to support both me and my dad for the past seven years, specifically two years for dad and the past five years with me.

Mom went with me to just about every doctor's appointment, as well as many of the chemo appointments, oncology appointments, and primary care visits. In addition, she was with me for every surgery, every Tampa trip, and every tough conversation with the doctors. She stayed at my house for surgery recovery, and she prepared meals and did basic housework during my incapacity. Mom was my advocate, supported my decisions, and encouraged me to continue with treatments, even on the days I wanted to give up, and she was my comforter. She never really complained about it. She passed up a few activities because of our doctor appointments or surgeries.

Brother, Anthony

My brother also helped out when he could. He called me on the phone, and came over occasionally to visit, but he knew not to get too close because I was immunocompromised. He did some of the housework and chores for me as well. He even gave me a tree of life plant, which is still going strong. Occasionally, he would dust and water the plants. His intentions were good, but he didn't completely understand that I couldn't have company at the risk of getting sick or ending up in the hospital. He would bring over my four-year-old niece for visits as well.

Lexi

We all know that children are germ carriers. This was not the best idea, but it was good to see her. This cute little blonde niece of mine didn't even want to come near me or look at me when I lost my hair. So I had to wear a wig whenever she came over. My brother was kind enough to shave his head for me as well. He also did this as a learning lesson for my niece. It did help her. As my hair started to grow back, she would feel my head and say: "It's like a baby bird"—meaning fuzzy. That was so cute. Still to this day, with my full head of hair, she touches my hair and says: "It's like a baby bird."

Michelle

Several of my friends offered to go grocery shopping for me. Some sent get-well wishes and cards of encouragement. Others called frequently, and others offered to visit. Michelle, who is just a year older than I am, offered to go grocery shopping for me. She and her husband spent a good two hours at the grocery store and managed to get everything on my list. There were a few phone calls to double-check on flavors and sizes, but this did save me a lot of time and energy. It also allowed me to get some house chores done on my own—it was a huge help to me. They also volunteered to watch my little dog, Shadow, several times when I had to go out of town.

The irony was that Michelle had just lost one of her close friends to cancer as well. Michelle herself had also suffered through breast cancer. She opted for a lumpectomy followed by radiation. We had the same breast surgeon and attended the same radiation clinic. These similar experiences also brought us closer together as friends. She is doing well with no complications.

Aubrey

Another friend of mine, Aubrey, offered several times to take me out. Aubrey is a few years younger than I am. She's a small business owner, married with children. She was going through a difficult time as well. Both of her parents and her sister-in-law were diagnosed with metastatic cancers. All of a sudden, cancer seemed to be very common in my town. With Aubrey's family members going through cancer and now her friend going through cancer treatments, she wanted to go out. This would serve as a small escape for a few hours, just to have a little fun, to be in a different environment, and to try to forget about cancer, and the devastation, and the toll it had taken on everyone.

For me, going out was a task in itself. I had to go when I wasn't tired, didn't feel nauseous, and was not immunocompromised. Aubrey also needed to find a babysitter, and then not be out too late. It took several months, but we did make the arrangements. We finally had a nice night out. For me, it was a break outside the house where I'd felt like a captive for so long. We organized with a few other people as well, and there were eight of us in total: Michelle and her husband, Aubrey and her husband, Aubrey's friend whom I'd met a few times prior, mom, and me. We did something fun. We went to the Escape Room. Several of us had never experienced it before, and we thought it would be something different. That it was. It was fun and exciting. Although we were together, we had space, so that was good. We worked together and escaped with one minute remaining.

After that hour in the Escape Room, we went to a sports bar for a bit. Yes, I felt "normal." I didn't feel sick; I felt the way a young woman should feel on a Friday night out: relaxed, enjoying the moment with friends, having a good time. Aubrey and I have since become closer since the death of all her family members who had cancer. She lost her sister-in-law in October 2019, her mom in November 2020, and then her dad in March 2020. That is hard to deal with—three deaths in six months. Yet, she was also there for me, texting, calling, and inviting me over. Actually, mom and I were invited to her house for Christmas dinner. It was a nice day out with good food, good conversation, and a nice time. Seldom did we get invited to dinner at anyone's house.

Elizabeth

Then there was Elizabeth. We go back about 20 years. She was also about 20 years older than I, and that was okay. We respected each other and worked around the same circle of people. We understood each other. We talked shop and shared our personal stories and craziness. Elizabeth was there from the beginning of my initial cancer diagnosis and took me to just about all my chemo treatments the second time around. We had code words for each other and the people working in the chemo center. We had "interesting," "floppy-hair girl," and "lunch" as our keywords. When we heard things that were controversial, "interesting" was the keyword. We didn't like "floppy-hair girl" too much, but she seemed to like me. Actually, one day she said: "I was the patient of the day." Wow! Shocker. Trust me.

I despised going to chemo, and I made this known. I didn't talk to anyone, and stayed in a corner by myself. Elizabeth had to wait in a small waiting room off the chemo room and was allowed to visit for only five minutes every hour It was there, or wait in the lobby waiting room. So, we would text each other back and forth and push the time limit. We saw no reason why Elizabeth couldn't sit next to me, and we chatted when the place was just about empty. But no. I think one time she was asked five times to go to the waiting room or come and get me later. Elizabeth drove an hour to pick me up, waited with me for four or five hours, took me to lunch, dropped me back at home, and then dropped me back at home. This was an all-day affair for her. She did this for me, without any complaints, and always offered to do more.

My mom appreciated this as well—it gave mom a break. Mom and Elizabeth are closer in age than Elizabeth and I are, and they have much else in common as well. They get along well, and sometimes we all go to lunch together. Elizabeth still sends me encouragement cards here and there, and we talk over the phone at least once a week to catch up. She has been there with me from the start and continues to be a strong supporter. She makes me laugh, tells me how it is, and will tell me if I am overreacting or just being stubborn.

Breezy

Then there was Breezy. Breezy is another female friend and former co-worker of mine in her late 60s. She had offered to drive me across the state on the four-hour ride to Tampa. Mom and I did take her up on this offer once. About an hour into our trip, a rock hit the windshield and cracked it. It was not that bad, but as we continued to drive, the crack spread from one side to the other. This was for a four-day surgery trip. Mom would stay with me two nights in the hospital, and Breezy had a friend who lived in Tampa, and whom she went to visit. After my discharge, we stayed two nights at a hotel before traveling back home. Breezy didn't mind the drive. I think she did mind that mom and I were fussy when we wanted food and she had to drive us. However, mom did pay Breezy for gas, food, and hotel. All in all, I knew I couldn't make the drive home after surgery, and mom didn't drive long distances or on highways, so we were fortunate to have Breezy with us on this trip.

Some other people would call and check in with me from time to time, offer to bring me things, or stop over for a quick visit. It was good to know that people cared and wanted to help. My neighbors would bring over a meal from time to time. Some brought me plants, get-well cards, and gift cards. I tried to keep my entire situation quiet. I told only a few close friends, some family members, and of course the human resources lady assigned to my case at work. Mom told her church group that I was sick and left it at that. The church group would send me healing cards and put me on their prayer list.

I was also on the prayer list with my direct sales company. I did direct sales as a side gig for two years, but I had to put it on hold with all this going on. I was impressed with the prayer department. One lady who was assigned to my case would call me about once a month to check in with me and see how I was doing. She wrote me get-well cards and even had the company send me flowers for surgery recovery—very nice and impressive. They are a biblically based company, and it showed. It was not about the product, it was about the people.

Sherry

Sherry, my friend and a higher-up with the direct sales company, would also text and visit and had me on the local direct sales prayer list as well. Sherry is my age, married, and works full time while also working her side gig (direct sales) part time. Sherry organizes our local direct sales team meetings and helped me with my side business during my downtime. She also respected my request and kept my situation quiet from the other team members. She kept me in the loop with what was going on with the company and thought of ways I could still make some money.

At this point, there was no income. My full-time teaching job ended due to my year-and-a-half sick leave absence. I had to basically give up my side gig, as I couldn't leave the house or be near people, and disability hadn't started yet. The bills were piling up due to all the surgeries, specialty doctors, chemo, radiation, the normal house bills, mortgage, and let's not forget about COBRA medical insurance, which was a must at $700 a month. I had to use most of my savings and emergency funds just to get through all this. Mom did give me a few dollars here and there, to get through a month or two, but that was it. The rest was up to me. It was a stressful time, and my medical oncologist recommended I join a cancer support group.

Support Groups

Overachiever that I was am, I joined two support groups. One was at the hospital for young ladies like myself (ages 45 and younger), which met once a month and was three towns over. The other one was in my town but was for all cancers, not just breast cancer. I would attend both when I could. I didn't feel that I really fit in at either group, but I kept going as I thought they would get better. But they never did really get better, and I didn't feel as though I related to anyone's story.

The monthly young adult group consisted of about eight women, who all had various stages of breast cancer. They had families, worked, and lost their jobs due to cancer as well. The only problem was that I thought these girls were wimps. Some opted for lumpectomy for their stage 0 breast cancer, and some opted for the double mastectomy, so that they could have better boobs. Others would sit there and cry and boo-who when they had a stage I breast cancer. Stage I is nothing. Yes, they had cancer, but it was small, contained, and required only a small surgery—no chemo, no radiation, nothing else but minor surgery and a few weeks of healing. So not for me. I had Stage III-C metastatic breast cancer that spread from my breast to my lymph nodes. I required major surgery, port insertion, chemotherapy, radiation, more surgery, and reconstruction. I felt that I was far worse off than these girls and didn't relate as they couldn't understand my situation with all the complications I had. This group was not really for me. I went to say that I went. I did talk to the facilitator about how I felt about that group, and she suggested I try another group.

I went to the metastatic cancer group twice and didn't really like it either. There was only one other person in this group, and that person was closer to death than I was. That made me feel sad, and why would I want to attend when this other lady had just a few months to live. I didn't want to get to know someone, only to have them die in a few months. However, I did feel that I had more in common with this lady than with the young girls. In this group, we did discuss the seriousness of metastatic cancer, how it would spread, and how we didn't want to prolong life just to comfort others. We actually talked about serious issues, such as our funerals arrangement, our dying wishes, Hospice, and our legacies. Finally, here was real, straightforward information, all the stuff that no one else wanted to talk about or hear about, but needed to be said. I stopped going after two visits due to my own radiation treatments and the inconvenience.

The other group I joined was a local cancer group in my town. This cancer group met weekly but was comprised mostly of senior citizens. I was the youngest member. I took mom with me a few times, as she was a cancer survivor and could possibly relate. This group had about a dozen active people who faithfully attended the weekly meetings. I think they met up mostly for social interaction, more than cancer support. Yes, they all had their stories of how cancer affected their lives, but no one was going through it the way I was. Great, so now I was with a bunch of seniors who couldn't relate to me because my surgeries were more modern and advanced than what their experiences were. Something else I didn't care for was they would end each meeting with a prayer. How can a public group take a religious stand? That should not be. Yes, many of the attendees were Christians, but this was open to the public. Many times I felt pressured into the prayer as I didn't feel like there was a chance for me to leave before they started. I'm not all into that. Don't pressure me. If you want to pray for me on your own time, which is fine, do it without me present, please. Mom and I did make friends with one lady there. She was in her 60s and had many health issues. She was the only one who would call or text to touch base. We occasionally met up for a meal and talked for a bit. That was it. No one else called, texted, or asked about us. So much for the support group. Yes, I know people are busy with their own lives, but still. If you are supposed to provide support, provide support. Anyway, I stopped going because I ended up in the hospital with sepsis and couldn't go out. So that was my out. Last I heard, the group had stopped meeting because of COVID-19, so that may be the end of it anyway.

All of these groups had one commonality. They were part of a very famous cancer society. This organization raised millions of donation dollars through walks, events, and drives. I previously supported this organization and participated in these events with mom. We even served as team captains for several years and helped raise hundreds of dollars for several of their fundraising campaigns. This organization also states that they provide rides to chemo treatment for patients and help with medical expenses and lodging while traveling for treatments or surgery. All I can say is my perspective has changed. I no longer support this organization in any way, shape, or form. I will not participate in any of their causes, events, or activities.

Several times, I asked the cancer organization for assistance with lodging expenses and was denied. I asked for medication assistance and was denied. I asked for a bill payment and was denied. Keep in mind that I asked on different occasions over three years and was denied every time. The excuses were: There is a six-week waiting list for lodging," "our system is down," and "we don't have a driver for the four-hour trip for you." And let's not forget: "That's a holiday week, we don't have availability." Like I had a say with scheduling an appointment around that holiday. The doctor's office is what scheduled it, I had an appointment card, but oh no, no accommodations available. So upsetting.

The only way to get free lodging was first to be on a waiting list, which was usually six to eight weeks out. Second, you had to stay in their lodge for at least six weeks during your treatment. In addition, there were no cleaning services, and you had to cook for yourself, clean for yourself, buy all your own supplies, share a kitchen, eat in the common kitchen area—not in your room—, watch TV only in the common room, not in your room, and be on lockdown from 8 p.m. to 8 a.m. What good was this? Oh, and no one could stay with you. Really? First off, if you are sick, why would you want to eat and watch TV with other sick people? Second, if I had the energy to cook, clean, and shop, why would I need to stay there? Third, why would I want to be alone with no help when I was that sick? This really didn't make any sense. Even the hospital had therapy dogs to come and visit the inpatients. Yes, it was across the hospital parking lot and convenient, but that was it. I got more service from a hotel. There I could eat in bed if I chose, order room service, or get food delivered. The hotel had a modern atmosphere, a cleaning service, and I even had the option to watch TV from the bed.

Yes, it was a struggle and an expense to go to Tampa for at least two days at a time every month. Gas, food, and hotels all add up. I had very little free time even to do anything when I was there. Mom and I tried a bed and breakfast once, but that didn't work. We booked a two-night stay, but left after night one. It turned out that we had rented a room with house privilege right next to the railroad track with a working train. Never again! It was a three-bedroom cottage not far from the specialty center, but it was on the "wrong side of the tracks"! The overall savings were not that great, either.

Our room was the master room with a private bathroom. Good thing, since the other bathroom, off the living room, was out of order. Our room had a double bed and a convertible ottoman to make a single bed. Mom, of course took the double bed. I rested on the ottoman. I say "rested" because the trains coming through at all hours of the night made certain that there was no sleep. The room had no cable, so watching TV was not an option. There were wires hanging from the exposed electrical sockets, broken blinds, and then there were the ants. Yes, I noticed a large ant pile right next to the double bed. It looked like the ants had burrowed their way through from outside the house to inside the bedroom. We didn't have any spray, so mom put shaving cream on them, and all along the baseboard of the entire wall with the bed. It actually worked! The ants died in the foam, and mom didn't get attacked by ants throughout the night. That was it— there was no way I was staying another night. No sleep, dusty blankets, no TV, other people renting out the other rooms—no thanks! I didn't care; we would drive home after my appointment and drive in the dark. It wasn't the safest idea, but it was better than going back to that rental house!

I usually had two or three appointments, either on the same day or over two days: one with the breast surgeon, the other with a medical oncologist, and then usually some type of test—blood work, MRI, or ultrasound. With the long drive, we would sometimes leave at 5 a.m. for the late morning appointments and other times leave at 8 a.m. for the late afternoon appointments. On the return, we would leave there at about 1 p.m. and get home at about 6 p.m. There really was not too much time for entertainment. We would have a nice dinner out, head for the hotel, and call it a night. I did manage to meet up with one of my friends for dinner twice during the entire year, and that was enjoyable.

Mom and I made a little routine. We found a few local places that would become our rest stops. We found a local restaurant that we enjoyed for lunch or early dinner, depending on our schedule. The portions were large, the prices were fair, and they even had tableside salad service. Both of us usually brought home leftovers. There really wasn't much to see during the hours on the country road, except for strawberry farms, a few cows here and there, and a stoplight. Sometimes we would go into a grocery store just to stretch our legs for a few minutes and take a break. Every trip had memory-making moments.

For all those who supported me during my difficult time, I thank you for your concern, phone calls, love, willingness to help, and friendship. There is no way I could have completed this difficult year of my life without your support. Mom, thanks you, too. Thank you for being there for her, giving her an outlet, providing her with comforting words, and listening to her about all the craziness cancer caused in our lives. Thank you for all the prayers, support, and well wishes for me and my family.

Cancer impacts the entire family, not just the patient. Every appointment causes anxiety. Every diagnostic test triggers the "what if" question. Every doctor walking into the exam room causes sweaty palms. Every difficult conversation brings tears to my eyes. However, knowing my family and friends are there for me helps alleviate these problems.

CHAPTER 6

The Funeral

Because I was so sick, difficult conversations were had with my family and doctors. Trust me, it was no easy task, thinking that every time I saw you or spoke to you it could be our last. I had seen my dad's slow decline with his metastatic cancer and felt the impact it made on me. I decided to have tough talks with my family and doctors. Since this was my second time going through Stage III-C cancer, I knew that my chances of getting healthy were slim. This was especially true if I didn't follow cancer treatment protocols: surgery, chemo, radiation, and medications. I did all of these as the doctors suggested, but I had a plan laid out in my cancer progressed to Stage IV.

The Tough Talks

If Stage IV were to occur—that is, cancer spread to lymph nodes, lungs, liver, bone marrow, or brain—I would not take treatment. I already had advanced, metastatic breast cancer as the cancer spread to 16 of my axillary lymph nodes, and also a contaminated lymph node in my upper chest area. Once this occurs and cancer travels within the body, chemo and radiation buy just a few extra months of life. I wanted quality of life versus quantity of life. I had watched dad choose quantity of life over quality, and I didn't agree with that. Why be chained to the doctor's office for daily treatments just to live a few extra months. I wanted to feel good, come and go, and not worry about immunity issues in my last few months of life.

I was prepared for these conversations. After dad's funeral, I expressed my thoughts to mom and my doctors. Mom said that whatever my wishes were, she would support me. The medical oncologist tried telling me that I would be making a mistake. The medications are out there to keep me alive. Why would I want to give up? But to me, I wasn't giving up—I'd fought this twice already. If my body was consumed by cancer, what was the sense? The result would be the same.

The Yellow Paper (DNR)

My primary care physician seemed to understand my reasoning and supported my decision as well. I did say that I would want comfort measures, but no cancer treatments, if the cancer should progress or return. I filled out a do not resuscitate (DNR) order, and my primary care physician signed it. My primary doctor was young, smart, and compassionate. She understood my situation, and agreed with my choices. She was open, honest, and straightforward—all the qualities I needed in a primary physician. The DNR was placed in my chart and put on file with the hospital as well. I keep the original on the front door of my refrigerator in case of an emergency. I have also brought it to all the hospitals where I've had surgery, just in case. This lets doctors know that if my heart should stop beating, they are not to perform any life-saving procedures, but should let me die naturally. I figure if my body and organs give out, then it is time to give in.

I told a few of my friends about this, and they didn't want to hear it. I wasn't trying to be morbid—I wanted to be realistic. And why not? Why wait for a critical situation to occur, where tough decisions need to be made? I could make my wishes known now, while I'm in my right mind and not under pressure.

I tried to express my desires to my brother, but he didn't want to hear of it. He said: "No one is dying—I don't want to talk about this. The tree of life is still going strong." From his mouth to God's ears! Yes, it is a very difficult situation to discuss, but it's a discussion that needs to be had. I want to be able to make decisions about my health as long as I can, and not put that burden on someone else to decide for me. I even went as far as having a revocable living trust made. This is a good thing to have, no matter the situation. I designated my assets, included my medical wishes, and assigned my belongings to others. I got a bit carried away, going around the house and attaching papers with names to objects I would like to pass down to others. I divided up, bagged, and labeled all my jewelry to be handed down as well. Stickers are still on the bottoms of many of my home decor pieces. It's fine with me. At least I know who gets what, and items will not be fought over.

Funeral Shopping

The hardest thing I did was shopping for my funeral. Yes, I shopped for my funeral. I started this just a few weeks after my dad's funeral. As I saw firsthand what I liked and didn't like about his. This was also just after my second right-sided mastectomy redo surgery, and just after my 44th birthday. I didn't think I would live to see 45, so I was out shopping for my funeral with hospital bands still on my wrist. Mom came with me. We started out where we had dad's service. I wanted a price for a prepaid funeral, a short remembrance service, followed by some food and drinks. I decided on more of a memorial service with my cremated ashes there. I didn't want to be laid out and have people touch my plastic-looking, cold, dead body.

All the funerals I'd attended in my life were like this, and I just hated them. I didn't want that. I wanted a quote for my service. I picked out my urn, Mass cards, registry book, flowers, songs, and photos. I thought the price this funeral home gave me was a bit high. I wasn't dead yet. I didn't need to make these decisions right then and there. I had some time to shop around, or so I hoped. I also thought that since we had just used this location for dad six weeks before, and mom had arrangements there, the price would be good. That was not the case. Off we went to another funeral home for comparison pricing.

It is really weird walking into a funeral home and planning your death. I went with this second funeral home, as I liked the options a bit better; they seemed to understand how I wanted the service and still offered food and beverages, as well as a nicer atmosphere. The package I picked had more photos, an upgraded urn, and a better insurance policy and payment plans than the first funeral home. I was kind of hoping the insurance policy would kick in, but that meant that I would have to die. I wasn't quite ready for that. If I should die before I finish paying the policy, all future payments would be written off. How nice was that? Perhaps, I would pay only six months of the three-year contract and not have my family worry about the rest of the expenses.

Well, here it is one year later, and I haven't died, and I'm still making those payments. Yes, I have all my songs picked out, my photos picked out and on a USB drive, and I have a picture board of my life ready for display. Not much else needs to be done. Hopefully, the "Theresa died" phone call will not be made for many years to come. I have made it to my 45th birthday and hope to make it another 45.

CHAPTER 7

What Dumbass Doctors Tell You: A Patient's Perspective

The following topics are things that my dumbass doctors told me and what my experience with it was:

"I Doubt It Is Anything"

Doctors need to listen to patients—yes, actually listen instead of forming their own conclusions about a diagnosis without having evidence. Women are taught from an early age to do regular breast self-exams, check for lumps, and report them or call the doctor with any changes. In my case, I did all of these, and when I went to the doctor with my concerns, I was told: "I doubt it is anything." I explained that I had found a small lump on a previous scar line that concerned me. I knew my body, knew my history, and knew the possibility of having cancer was high. I was told over and over again: "It is most likely scar tissue, and don't worry."

Why not err on the side of caution and just say: "Well, let's take a biopsy and wait for the results." Nope. The doctor convinced me that I was overreacting and there was no need for a biopsy. I listened to the doctor when the reply was "I doubt it is anything, most likely scar tissue." With anxiety and worry that there was a possible chance of cancer and months of complaining, I actually convinced the doctor that a biopsy was warranted on this area of concern that was now getting larger.

Well, let me tell you, that scar tissue is not going to start forming into a lump after two years. Every piece of my being was telling me that this was a new lump, not scar tissue buildup, and it was something to worry about. Mom always told me: "If someone says not to worry, it is time to worry!" Mom is usually right.

As I was lying on the table, I asked the doctor: "Please go longer and wider to be sure there are no margins left, and the entire specimen comes out." I was assured this was a simple procedure, everything was out, and told not to worry. Here we go again with the "don't worry." Panic and worry started to set in. The doctor assured me and mom, who was in the waiting room, that I was just overreacting. Again, he said: "Most likely it is nothing to worry about." Again, why would he say this without knowing the status for sure? I was just about convinced it was nothing.

Well, 10 days later, mom and I went back to the office for the biopsy results. I was right, and the doctor was wrong. I had something to worry about—the diagnosis. It was exactly what I was worried about: cancer. Why would a physician make a diagnosis and say "Don't worry, I doubt it's anything," without having actual evidence? I don't know. Perhaps the God complex? Listen to the patient. Patients do know their bodies. While I understand physicians are there to reassure the patients about possible outcomes, they should be saying: "Let's wait and see how the pathology comes back, and then we can discuss further." The cancer diagnosis was more of a surprise to the physician than to me. Was this a lesson learned for the physician? I hope so, but that God complex can get in the way.

This is one of the reasons why I decided to go to the specialty center. The doctor didn't listen to me. How could I trust a doctor who didn't take me or my health seriously? What if I had not been so persistent? What if I had continued to see this doctor? What if I had let it go? Would this cancer have been found early enough for treatment, or would it have been be too late? It's true that I have anxiety about my health, but I think I have good reason for that. I have had so many complications, side effects, and procedures that I can't help but be anxious. Doctors, especially breast surgeons, need to understand that, and listen to the patient.

"Cancer Doesn't Hurt"

I have heard myself many times in my life that when there is a bruise, lump, or bump, if it doesn't hurt, it is not cancer, so don't worry about it. For the most part, this is true. Most cancers don't hurt at first. However, some cancers can hurt, and they often manifest as a painless lump, bump, bruise, or some other symptom, such as coughing or bleeding. The problem with hearing that most cancers don't hurt is that many potential issues can be overlooked. I found this to be true. The more advanced cancers, like my own Stage III-C breast cancer situation, have the potential to cause pain.[1]

Cancer pain can come from different areas. It sounds simple, but sometimes that pain is actually caused by the cancer itself. When cancer grows and harms nearby tissue, pain can be generated. You may also feel a tight muscle pain or experience headaches that have nothing to do with cancer. Pain is an indication that something is wrong in the body. It can be a sign that cancer has already spread within the body. Sometimes, pain can be an early symptom of bone cancer or testicular cancer. Pain should not be ignored. Many people experience back pain. However, this can be an indication of colon, rectal, pancreatic, or ovarian cancer. Others may complain of a headache that doesn't go away and may have brain cancer.

Cancer pain can be an indication of:

- Tumor growth compression on nearby structures.

- The spread of cancer to other body parts or organs.

- Cancer that has spread to the bones, also known as bone metastases. Bone cancer is known to be very painful. To help with pain control, some medications may be used. However, bone metastases are usually treated with radiation therapy. Sometimes, bone-modifying medications may be initiated.[4]

- Tumor secretions: Some cancers and tumors secrete proteins that can cause pain. This is seen often in patients who have either small-cell lung carcinoma or squamous cell lung cancers.[4]

- Nerve pain: Nerve pain, sometimes referred to as neuropathic pain, may be caused by the pressure of a tumor on nerves. This is a common occurrence for chemotherapy patients who are on medications, such as Taxol, and radiation therapy. This causes pain and numbness in the fingers, hands, feet, and toes, which is also known as peripheral neuropathy.

In my case, my whole situation started with some intermediate, sharp pain in the biceps region of my right arm. At first, I thought it was just a muscle strain and decided to wait a few weeks to see if it got better. Well, it only got worse. Life went on. In the meantime, I had a mammogram that showed dense breasts. There was a recommendation for follow-up with ultrasound. The ultrasound was scheduled and completed, and the results were negative. However, my arm pain increased in frequency, and over the next two months pain started to radiate up into the side of my right breast. I went to see a breast surgeon just to be safe. He ordered a breast MRI. I was told: "I doubt it's anything, but let's get one just to make sure it's nothing." Good thing this MRI was ordered as the results showed positive for breast abnormality. Now the MRI report recommended a breast biopsy be done. The breast biopsy was completed via an outpatient stereotactic procedure. (This procedure is done under "twilight," meaning that the patient is awake but consciously sedated.)

Now, stressed about all the recommendations, I had to wait for the results. This was very stressful and made me anxious. One Friday morning, while I was at work at 8:45 a.m., I got "the call." The words I had suspected, but didn't want to hear—"You have cancer"—came across the phone lines.

This was followed by: "I'll see you in the office next week to discuss further. Good-bye." Ugh! Did I mention that this call was received at work on a Friday morning? Now what? How was I supposed to start the workday being productive, and not worry about it over the weekend? Seriously?

"Lose Weight"

Weight loss should be the least of most medical oncologists' concerns. One doctor told me that his goal for me was weight loss. Yes, while I may be overweight, weight loss during a cancer diagnosis was not my biggest concern. The cancer and the cancer treatments themselves will usually cause weight loss—not only weight loss but muscle loss too. Cancer treatments will also cause extreme fatigue. There was no need to purposefully go on a diet now! Dumbass doctor! Didn't he know the body produces cytokines? Cytokines are the body's own chemical substances that can lead to weight loss, muscle loss, and a decrease in appetite.[5] I believed my main goal should be my cancer status, not weight loss. Are the cancer treatments working? Am I getting better or worse? What are the next steps? Not weight loss.

Weight loss also usually occurs naturally from the side effects of radiation and chemotherapy. This is due to the lack of appetite, reduced calorie consumption, and treatment side effects, such as nausea, vomiting, and mouth sores. All these factors can affect your ability to eat normally, contributing to weight and muscle loss. Muscle loss also plays a part in weight loss due to fatigue. A decreases in exercise and other physical activities will also contribute to weight and muscle loss.[5]

Healthy eating tips for women undergoing treatment for breast cancer include:

- Eat a rainbow and variety of fruits and vegetables (unless you're on a neutropenic diet).

- Try new foods, even things you didn't like before, as they may taste good during cancer treatment.

- Eat high-protein and lean meat. Soy is a controversial topic.

- Limit animal products that are high in fat.

- Bake or broil foods rather than frying.

- Choose fat-free or low-fat dairy products.

- Drink plenty of fluids to stay hydrated, but avoid sugary drinks, such as soda. (Check with your doctor if you have a fluid restriction.)[7,8]

Studies have suggested that exercise can help lessen side effects, such as pain, nausea, and fatigue from chemotherapy. However, each patient should check with their doctor to understand any exercise restrictions that might be appropriate for their case. Exercise or physical therapy may be prescribed after surgery to help the patient regain arm mobility and strength. Be aware that any surgery to the breast, underarm, and lymph nodes can impact the range of motion of the arm, shoulder, and chest. Physical therapy exercises can help aid in the restoration of function and help improve flexibility. Women should talk to their doctor before beginning any new exercise routine. Ask if a referral to a physical or occupational therapist is recommended. At first, these exercises will be explained and supervised. Some will be home exercises that will be done on a regular basis to help prevent muscle loss and increase range of motion. Some exercises can begin a few short days after surgery, while other movements should be avoided until after any drains or stitches have been removed.[4]

After speaking to a registered dietitian and licensed nutritionist, my outcome was that I should eat whatever and whenever I wanted to eat. If you want a milkshake, by all means have it. Don't deprive yourself. Cancer patients need calories. The best eating plan for a cancer patient is one that consists of frequent small meals throughout the day—three main meals and about two snack meals.

Do you think I'm going to be concerned about my diet and losing weight while I'm worried about cancer, the lab results, the upcoming test, test results, trying to keep a family together, cleaning the house, going grocery shopping, and having a life? Do I need to worry about weight loss on top of all this? Plus, as already mentioned, weight loss is going to occur naturally just due to cancer itself.

Also, depending on the lab results, a neutropenic diet may be recommended. This is a diet in which fresh, raw fruits and vegetables are cut from the diet because of lab values and immunity issues. So, in essence, if these food are cut from the diet, more carbs, such as bread and cake, and greater quantities of food are substituted, and weight gain can occur. It is a very hard balance not to add excessive calories without exercise because weight gain will occur.

For me, the chemo weeks were my diet weeks. Thanks to chemotherapy, I ate only between 500 and 800 calories a day. This was due to a lack of appetite, feeling of nausea, and being tired. During the chemo weeks, my weight would drop between 5 and 8 pounds. During my off-chemo weeks, my weight would then increase 5 to 10 pounds due to an increase in food consumption. It was also hard being on a neutropenic diet in the summer while I was on chemo. The only fruits allowed were oranges and bananas, after the skins were scrubbed and then peeled. So much for enjoying all the summer fruits, such as peaches, berries, grapes, and watermelon. I love summer fruits. I even attempted eating a strawberry—bad decision. I broke out in a rash from it, so no other fruit besides oranges and bananas. I decided just to not eat those at all.

"Stay Away From Dr. Google"

At many of my doctor's visits, I asked questions about my "situation." Where did I get some of these questions? The Internet, of course. You have seen them before: "Questions To Ask Your Doctor," "What You Should Be Discussing With Your Physician," "How To Get The Most Out of a Doctor's Visit," and so on. I did my due diligence. I went to reputable sites, looked up a few articles, and also came up with some of my own questions. I even looked up some recent studies to confront the doctors with. Well, that did not sit well with the dumbass doctors. The dumbass doctors weren't aware of the studies, couldn't answer my questions, or tell me any percentages of treatment prognosis. Their answer to me was: "Stay away from Dr. Google and off the Internet."

What happened to patients being well informed about their condition? I had one doctor tell me he had to go and look up the answer to my question. I said: "Fine, I'll wait."

He came back to the office with a book, flipped to a page, and said: "Your answer is in this chart." I asked if I could see it; he said "No," closed the book, and walked out. What a faker! Did he think I was going to buy that line? He just picked any page and gave me a dumbass answer. Mom and I got up and checked out. No, I never went back to see that dumbass doctor! Sorry, if a doctor can't be honest with me, I don't want him treating me.

While I understand the need to look up some info, it can be a stressor. It can create anxiety and allow patients to jump to conclusions. However, the patient wants and needs answers now. Is this detrimental? Are the results good or bad? What can this mean? The Internet can provide peace of mind. Anxiety builds when a patient has test results and doesn't have a follow-up visit for a week. By the way, did you ever notice that most results come back on Fridays? Ever try calling the office for answers on a Friday? Messages are taken, and there's no return call until late Monday or Tuesday. That is if you even get a call back. At the same time, patients should be well informed of their condition, be active in the care plan, and be able to discuss options with their physicians.

As for me, my labs were drawn on a Tuesday and sent off. Healthcare technology is wonderful with having notifications in your email when your labs are back. However, for me this was my worst nightmare. Of course, as soon as the email came in at 12:15 p.m. on a Friday, I was on the lab patient portal within minutes. What are the results? Better? Worse? Am I dying? Am I going to live? Log in, get results, compare from the last lab, trend my results, and right back to Google I go. The search title includes "What does an elevation in cancer markers mean"? How to lower cancer markers? What is the reliability of the test? And so on. More on cancer tumor markers later. Besides, the patient gets the results before the doctor has seen them, so there's no sense calling the doctor and asking: "Can you explain the results to me?"

The response is: "We didn't get them back yet," or "The doctor hasn't signed off, so call back on Monday."

Ugh, the anxiety builds. Google said elevation means cancer. Great, now I'm dying! Perfect timing too, just in time for the weekend! Then at 3:30 p.m. on Friday, perhaps the doctor's office calls and says: "Your blood work came back, and the doctor says everything is good."

I ask, "How can it be good if the levels are higher than last time?"

The answer: "You can discuss at your next visit." My next visit is not for another week. The doctor said my labs are good. Now, back to worrying over the weekend and starting "the list" for the next office visit. Blood test results? Why are the levels up? What does this mean? Are we going to retest? If so, when? How long for the results? What if the results show the levels are up again? It's a never-ending cycle of anxiety, fear, and worry.

While one in three Americans uses the Internet to research health information, Googling can cause added stress and anxiety.[6] If you aren't careful about where you're getting your information, you might end up with the wrong information. Here are some guidelines to avoid misleading or inaccurate information.[6]

- Use only reputable websites, such as government agencies, health organizations, or academic centers.

- Be sure the information is current. Cancer care, recommended treatments, and survival rates are constantly changing.

- Discuss your findings with your healthcare team and address any questions or concerns you have.

"Tumor Markers Mean Nothing"

In addition to the regular every-two-weeks blood draws, the standard complete blood count (CBC), and complete metabolic panel (CMP), my monthly tumor markers were also obtained. The tumor markers were the CA 15-3 and CA 27.29, both specific to breast cancer. The tumor markers measured the status of disease progression, and the effects of chemotherapy. The CBC was drawn before the chemo treatment, with results within

10 minutes of the draw. The CMP was sent to the lab, and results would be provided at the next visit with the doctor. Cancer antigen 15-3 (CA 15-3) is used to determine the chemo response related to the breast cancer treatments. It also projects the percentage of disease recurrence.[16] The CA 27.29 monitors how much antigen is in the blood. These tests are limited to the following two functions: monitoring the progression of metastatic breast cancer and monitoring the treatment of the cancer.[16]

The lower the values the better because this means the treatment is working and the values correspond to a positive treatment response. An increase in value indicates the cancer is advancing and the treatments are not working.

These specimens were sent to the lab, and I was alerted by email when the results were available. The first time I received an email from the lab, I was surprised. I had the blood draw, but I was not informed that the blood was going to the lab or that these tests were ordered. So of course, from then on, I asked what tests were being performed. What was going to the lab? When would the results be back? When I saw the email from the lab, of course I had to log on and get my results. The results were initially similar to the previous ones, so all was good. Learning that everything was the same brought peace of mind.

The second month, I was again alerted by email that results were ready. I logged in, and this time the results were still in range, but elevated. This was also after chemo treatment number two out of four. So, why were the numbers going up? Was the chemo not working? Was something else going on? Was there more disease progression? These were questions I wanted answers to.

So, of course, I went to Google to see what I could find. Most of what I found was that elevation means the disease is progressing, the cancer is getting worse. Panic started to set in when I read: "These markers tend to increase whenever cancer is present." That was what my results were showing—an increase in values. So, I went to the doctor's office, asked to speak to someone about my test results, and was added to the nurse practitioner's schedule. When my name was called, I was vitalized, roomed, and sat and waited for what seemed like a lifetime before the nurse practitioner entered. When she saw me there, she said she tried to call me about my results two times and got no answer. I asked her what number she called because my phone didn't ring.

She proceeded to tell me that my labs were "fine." Fine? How can this be? I understood my values were in range, but they had doubled in value. Initially, the CA 15-3 had been 10, and now it was 20, and the range was <32. And the CA 27.29 had been 19, and now it was 33, and the range was <36. What did this indicate? Did it mean that the chemo was ineffective? Was the cancer getting worse and spreading?

These numbers were not fine. When I had cancer the first time, my levels were in range at 15 and 16, respectively. Now they were higher, and they were "fine"? The nurse practitioner left the room and stated she would be back. A few minutes later she returned with another person. I asked again, straight out: "Is the chemo working or not?" The reply was that this was the office manager, and she was here to be a witness to what the nurse practitioner was about to say.

I thought to myself: "Oh great, here it comes, the words I really don't want to hear. Am I prepared for this?"

But the nurse practitioner said: "I spoke to the doctor, and she said all is fine. I don't know what more to tell you." Then the office manager stated that she had heard that I had been rude to the office staff. She didn't give me any details about dates, times, or examples, but she said my attitude could not continue. It was up to me if I wanted to come back and complete treatment.

"If not, that is fine because there are probably 20 other people who want the chemo chair," she told me. I was shocked—this was not what I was expecting to hear at all. I said I would be back in a few days to continue with chemo. I left the office feeling attacked, and I still didn't get the answers about why my markers were elevated. I felt that the chemo was not working, the disease was progressing, and the office was a money-making business.

Then I did the next best thing. I got a copy of my labs and sent them off via email for review at a specialty oncology department at an educational research facility. Of course, it was a Friday afternoon, and I was not expecting to hear back until the following week, but I felt a sense of relief knowing that I would get some answers soon. Monday came, and there was an email regarding my results. The doctor said the results were okay, and not to worry. "Tumor markers mean nothing, and the institute hasn't used them in over 10 years." In addition, they are "nonreliable, outdated tests that often show false positives."

This doctor suggested scans and diagnostic tests be ordered to find out what was happening. Ah, an answer! That was all I wanted. Scans: perfect! Now, more questions: If these tests are outdated, why are they still being used and ordered by the doctors (going back to my "money-making business" thought process)? Why did I get a bill from the lab for more than $900 for them? These tests caused me nothing by aggravation, stress, and worry, not to mention lots of money. I asked my local doctor not to order them anymore.

"Radiation Only Takes Five Minutes"

"Don't worry, you will be in and out in five minutes." "The setup takes longer than the treatment." Those were some of the phrases I heard when it came to radiation. Well, BS on that! Perhaps these statements are true for 3D conformal radiation, but not for me. I had intensity modulated radiation therapy (IMRT). I was lying on the table for 30 to 40 minutes per session, Monday through Friday, and was scheduled for more than 30 treatments. For the past 19 sessions, my skin just got a little bit red, like a sunburn—nothing major. A few drops of aloe, and all was better.

Treatment 20 was where my problem started. I woke up the next day, Saturday, with radiation blisters. By Sunday, I had a streak of vertical blisters on the side of my chest, with an 8 out of 10 on the pain scale. Cool showers didn't help too much. Padding, slight compression, and not moving helped the most. I lay in bed most of the day. Monday morning was the next treatment. I stopped at the front desk to check and said I was in a lot of pain and was blistered. The receptionist told me to go ahead to the treatment area. As I walked by the nurses' station, I told the nurse the same thing. She asked me to change into a gown, and she would come and check my skin. Of course, my radiation oncologist was not in that day, but an associate was. When the nurse checked my skin, she saw the line of blisters, snapped a few photos, and contacted my doctor. I was to see the associate doctor for this, and then decide if treatment was going to happen that day or not.

An associate doctor came in and took a look. She was trying to rule out shingles. I told her it was not shingles, but radiation burn blisters. If it was shingles, they would have been spread throughout my trunk area and on my back. This was not the case. Another dumbass possible diagnosis from yet another "medical professional." After some convincing, she agreed with me and said it was radiation burn. I got a prescription for Bliss Cream and proceeded with radiation treatment. The plan was to check in with my radiation oncologist tomorrow, prior to radiation treatment, to see if treatment needed to be halted or if it was a go. I was on a time deadline. I needed to continue with radiation as much as possible. I had to complete all 33 treatments before the end of the month. My next scan was planned, along with port removal in three weeks. I was not delaying these procedures!

The next day came, and I went in early to see the doctor before treatment. He was convinced that I did have shingles, and again I disagreed and told him that I blistered when I got a bad sunburn. That didn't go over well, and I was prescribed an antiviral, to treat the shingles, and pain medicine. There was to be no treatment for the next three days. Well, if it was shingles, now I felt that they (the medical professionals) didn't want me to contaminate anything, as I was contagious. It was a nice, welcome change to know that I didn't need to get up early and go to treatment for the next few days—something of a return to normalcy.

The blisters and pain increased over the next few days. On the fourth day, I went back in to see the doctor. The pain was a 9 out of 10 on the scale, my blood pressure was 150/100, and yes, I was hurting. With my skin sloughing off and oozing, it was another week without treatment. At this point, I was fine with this decision. I needed to heal my skin in the next 10 days, so I could go to the operating room for port removal. I even had the chance to sleep in up until 11 a.m., as the pain medicine took a toll. I took it every four or five hours, and then slept for a good two or three hours afterward. The doctor also suggested I refill the Bliss Cream. That was not going to happen. It cost $65—not covered by insurance—, and it was a small container that didn't even seem to make a big difference. Don't even get me started on how being sick can make a person go broke!

At this point, I needed to wait the extra week, so the blister could dry up. The skin needed to heal before I could continue with radiation. My port removal surgery was just a few days away. Everything was set: Surgery was confirmed, the hotel reservation was confirmed, and the dog sitter was confirmed. If it was suggested that the entire radiation needed to be re-started because of the blister outbreak, my answer was no way! I'd take my chances! I just had to take two weeks off due to burns and possible shingles. I'd had 22 treatments. You can't tell me the 22 treatments meant nothing. Of course it did something—just take a look at my chest—my skin was peeling off, raw skin was exposed, and many areas were red are weeping.

For me, radiation caused complications. All this rawness, weeping, and redness caused me to be very sick, with nausea, vomiting, chills, and fever. It was so bad that I went to the ER. I was admitted for treatment of sepsis due to cellulitis, due to radiation burns. (Read more about this in Chapter 4, recounting my hospital visit.)

All I know is that radiation took a major toll on my body. I was starting to realize that the radiation was doing something. There was no way radiation did nothing. Let's also remember that it is all on the outside of my skin. What did it do to the inside of my chest, lungs, and neck? Most likely it fried everything up. Now I have a better understanding why most doctors say you should wait at least six months after radiation before getting any type of surgery in the area.

The "five-minute" treatment didn't come until the last two weeks of treatment, called "boost." This is where the area was treated more superficially, and treatment was more localized. Yes, then I was in and out in five minutes. It was still the same, lying in the mold, but this time I was able to breathe normally, and the machine was on for only 20 seconds. Positioning was what took the longest, and the treatment was fine. It took fifteen minutes from walking in the door to treatment to getting dressed and walking out the door. If all the treatments had been like that, I wouldn't have minded . . . as much.

"Radiation Is Like Going Tanning"

I have never been in a tanning bed, but I don't think radiation is anything like tanning. For one, I know when a person goes tanning, they wear a swimsuit. I don't think they go in the tanning bed topless, or do they? With radiation, you are placed in a mold, told not to move, and you lie on a table in a cold room with a machine that moves around you. There's no music, nothing to look at, and you're bored out of your mind. The only thing you can do to pass the time is to count the ceiling tiles and listen to yourself breathe. I got good at figuring out where I was in my session by the number of breaths I took during the radiation. After the first two breaths and the machine going around, the therapists would come in and place a warm towel over me and call it the "spa treatment." This was to create a layer between the machine and my skin to protect my internal organs from the strong radiation beam. Yes, it felt good, but when I was lying on a cold table half naked, I'm sure anything would be a welcome comfort measure. After they left the room, I would have to hold my breath seven more times, for at least 30 seconds per breath—holding and allowing the machine to spin around each time before my session would end. I think the only similarity to tanning is that you come out red!

"You Will Have A Slight Sunburn"

Another lie! Don't believe it for a minute. My experience was that I ended up with second-degree burns: painful blisters, chest redness, peeling, and cracked skin that seeped and oozed sticky, clear serous fluid. While I put burn cream, aloe vera, hydrocortisone cream, prescription Bliss Cream, and lidocaine gel over all these open burns, I had more than a slight burn.

I also covered the area with nonstick gauze. I had to become a bit creative with taping anything to my skin. I have an adhesive allergy and get blisters from tape. For a few days, I lay in bed without moving. I was able to hold the nonstick gauze in place for an hour, then change it, as it would be soaked through. Two days later, I came up with the idea of using maxi pads to absorb the seepage and using the "glue" side to stick to the inside of my shirt. This was a good idea that worked well. Still, every few hours I needed to repeat the process, as the drainage soaked through. I was cautious and kept my arm near my chest to help ensure I didn't lose a maxi pad. Can you imagine one falling out of my shirt during a grocery run? Oh my God! No, thanks. Imagine if someone noticed and said: "Honey that is not where it goes."

My skin and blisters were red. I could feel the topical heat. Blisters were coming out within hours. My chest felt like it was on fire. The pain was so bad that I had to take prescription opioids just to take the edge off. I took a picture of the area, as I felt this was more than "just a slight sunburn." Does this look like a slight sunburn to you or something more?

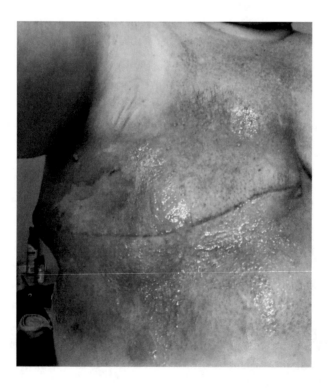

Let's just say that if it was a slight sunburn, would the doctor stop treatment for nine days to allow for healing to occur? I think not. I have had a severe sunburn before, and I blistered. This was yet another reason why I didn't think I had shingles. Shingles do not come and go within two weeks. They linger up to six weeks. Funny—I stopped radiation, and the blisters calmed down. That would not happen if I truly had shingles. These doctors! I tell you that these are all real and true experiences. The medical professionals make everything sound like it is no big deal—all lies. If they told the truth, I think a lot more people would opt out. After all, they are in business to make money, right? What happened to helping people?

"Left-Sided Port"

Port surgery should be no big deal either. This is a very common outpatient procedure that many cancer patients get for chemotherapy treatment. In preop, I was told I would be having a left-sided port placed for chemotherapy. All was good, or so I thought. What was there to worry about? Everything was going smoothly. The medical team understood the procedure. I signed all the paperwork. Then, just before I was taken to the OR, I was asked: "Do you want to be sedated?" What the heck? Of course. Did they think I wanted to be awake while the doctor cut into my chest, put needles into my neck, and sutured me up? What kind of stupid question was that—did I want sedation? Who goes through surgery without sedation? Like I needed this stress, just before going into the OR. Sedation was good, I woke up in recovery and had no idea that the surgery had taken place. Perfect!

The nurse allowed mom to come back and sit with me. She then proceeded to go over home care instructions. She told me to go easy, and not to wash the right side of my chest for a day. No shower, no lifting, and no bending. Wait, what? Did she say "the right side"? Oh, yes she did. I was told I was supposed to have a left-sided port, so why did I have it on the right side? I tried to feel around, and sure enough it was on the opposite side. I had a fit. How did that happen? All the paperwork stated "left side." I had verbal confirmation in preop that it was left side. Now, I woke up, and it was on the wrong side.

"Call the doctor!" I yelled. "Take me back to the OR and take it out. It's wrong! It had to be on the left, as the right side is my surgery side, and it can't be there for surgery."

The doctor took it upon himself to do a right-sided port because he said my veins were "torturous." Why hadn't he come to get consent from my mom first, to see if the right side was an option? Who was he to decide to change the order? Why didn't he call the breast surgeon who wrote the order? Dumbass doctor! Anyway, the port was there to stay, and the surgery would now be postponed until after chemo was completed (months from now). No thanks to this dumbass doctor! Well, guess what? Turns out I was allergic to the port. It was in for only a week, had to be removed, and, with a new doctor, I had a left-sided port!

"Margins Are Clear"

Clear margins on examination are the goal of any pathology. Biopsies are done to determine whether tissue is cancerous or noncancerous. These procedures can be done in the office, surgical center, or hospital. I have come to learn not to trust initial pathology reports of clear margins. The final pathology report is what is most important. The initial report is just that: a report at the time of tissue removal. The final report comes a few days later, after a microscopic exam of the tissue to see if anything has grown or progressed. This is the real report. I have had two instances where the initial report was clear, and the final showed positive margins. Usually, initial and final reports show the same result, and that is fine.

It just shocks me every time the initial is clear and the final is positive. When I hear "clear margins," that is good news. I heave a sigh of relief and feel a release of stress and lower anxiety. I have a sense of being healthy. Then, I get the bad news, that final pathology showed positive margins. That means more surgery to remove the unhealed wound from two weeks ago. Then, the anxiety builds again. Another surgery. How many times do I need to go through this? Does it ever end?

"No Follow-up Needed"

I longed for the days when I would hear "No follow-up needed." To me, this means no need to come back, all is well, and so are you. I would have freedom from doctor appointments, no more tests, and a chance to live life to the fullest and not worry about my health. I heard the words and thought it would be good. Well, not exactly. The meaning was not what I thought. The real meaning was: "You are a very unique patient, and we just don't know what else to do for you."

"Unique" is a term I heard from many of the doctors. What made me so unique? Was I an alien? Was it because I was so unique they couldn't figure me out? Was it that I knew my body and listened to it when the doctors didn't? Was it because I was an educated patient who asked questions? Was it because all I wanted was a doctor who would have a conversation about my health and not dictate what they wanted from me? Was it because I had already played the "what if" game and had a plan? Or was it because I was terminal and there was no money to be made from me? Or because these doctors were not up to date and didn't want to be questioned by me any longer? Was it a God complex? Was it because they were dumbass doctors? I was a bit disappointed after my initial expectations, but I guess in the long run it was still a "good" outcome. The doctors didn't want to see me, and I didn't want to see them.

CHAPTER 8

Advocate for Yourself

What have I learned from all my medical issues? The major lesson was that you need to be your own patient advocate. What does that mean? According to the National Cancer Institute, a patient advocate is one "who helps patients communicate with their healthcare providers so they get the information they need to make decisions about their health-care."[20] A patient advocate gives the patient an opportunity to voice their opinion, have their needs met, and maintain a level of control. This can be a designated person or the patient. In my case, I self-advocated. I spoke up for myself.

What steps did I take to ensure I had the correct information? I was not afraid to ask questions. If a physician feels challenged or intimidated by you asking questions, my advice is to get a new doctor. You can even get a second opinion. Doctors are there to guide you, provide recommendations, and give you options through open, honest, transparent, and respectful conversations. Do not allow doctors to dictate or pressure you into a decision. Remember, doctors are not God. Ultimately, your health is your decision. Sometimes compromise is best. Do your own research. You have options about your health. The face-to-face time with the provider is usually very short—maybe 15 minutes. Make a list of your questions to stay on track. Cross them off as you get the answers.

I also had a second set of ears with me at each appointment. Usually, it was mom, but sometimes Elizabeth. This lends itself to further discussion and concerns not only while in the office, but afterward as well.

Next, keep your own records. It is your health. You are entitled to have copies of all your records. Office notes, diagnostic test results, lab tests, and pathology results all belong to the patient. You may need to sign a release to get a copy, but get them. If you have access to a patient portal, review them in the portal. If something is not right, ask to have it amended. You have a right to know that the information in your chart is accurate. By keeping a copy of your medical information, you can compare results, know the dates when you had certain tests, and track your progress. I used a spreadsheet for weekly lab results to track immunity levels. A patient portal also works because many of them allow you to track your labs over time.

All these steps lead to patient empowerment. It is important to be as empowered as possible. This provides a sense of control as well. Some of my doctors told me that I drive the bus, and they choose to get on or get off. Meaning, that I was in control. The number of passengers didn't matter. I would get to the next stop with or without them on board. This is a pretty good analogy, don't you think? The providers could recommend and suggest certain things, but it was up to me to accept them or not. For example, they could tell me to drive the speed limit. If I accepted this statement, I wouldn't get a speeding ticket. If I didn't take the suggestion, I may or may not get pulled over and issued a citation. Was that a chance I wanted to take? For safety reasons, I agreed to drive the speed limit.

Keep in mind that the providers are providing recommendations. They are just that: recommendations. Their advice does not necessarily have to be followed. In addition, the consequences of our actions need to be considered and weighed. For example, I am not taking hormone blocker agents. Yes, there is a higher chance of recurrence. If I should get cancer again, I will need to assume responsibility for my actions. Now, I'm sure I will question whether it was because I didn't take the medication. Would the cancer have come back regardless? At least I have a sense of control over the situation. It is an acquired skill, but with practice, self-advocacy becomes easier.

At first, it may be easier to be someone else's advocate. Helping others advocate for themselves empowered me to be a stronger advocate for myself.

I used my previous experiences to help others in situations similar to mine. During the last five years of my cancer battle, I have had three friends who also had breast cancer. They all reached out to me for advice, since they knew my story. Actually, one of them even suggested I write this book.

I told each of them the same things: Ask questions of your doctors. Do your own research. Get a second opinion. We all had the commonality of having breast cancer, but I didn't want them to experience complications, as I did. I was trying to pay my experiences forward. Share words of encouragement, provide support, and be a good listener and a good friend.

One of these people had Stage I cancer, and the local breast doctor—the same one I had—suggested a double mastectomy. She didn't really like that option when her cancer was small, contained, and easily removable. She thought a lumpectomy was a better option for her. I provided her the name and phone number of the specialty center four hours away, and she was glad she went. While she also thought it was a long drive, she knew it was worth the trip.

The specialty center recommended a lumpectomy, and that is what she had. No additional treatments such as radiation or chemotherapy were suggested, and she is doing relatively well. She does have some lymphedema in her arm, but that is typical for breast cancer patients. She is grateful to me for having suggested a second option, provided her with research, and paid it forward.

Another friend of mine had more aggressive breast cancer with recurrence, like me. Her initial treatments included a lumpectomy, radiation, and chemotherapy. She was cleared for about two years, and then had a recurrence. She went through the same procedures again: another port, another surgery, more chemo, more radiation, and of course more tests. The only problem was that this time she was Stage IV. The breast cancer metastasized to her liver. She is having a hard time with the chemo this time. For some reason, both of us experienced many more side effects with chemo on our second go-arounds. I have been there to provide guidance, support, and friendship. I mail her greeting cards and care packages and call at least once a month, just to check in with her. During difficult times, we need to support each other and advocate for others, as well as ourselves.

CHAPTER 9

Where Are We Now?

The Last of the Surgeries

It has been four years since my cancer diagnosis, and it has been a hard journey. I am just starting to see a ray of hope drawing near. I have been feeling well since I completed my radiation treatments. I even have a certificate of radiation completion to prove it. My last treatment was just over six months ago. My skin is all healed up, and the hyperpigmentation is just about faded. I do still have some rib pain, but no one knows why.

This pain did start after about the third week of treatment and has only intensified. The radiation physician is stumped. At first, he said it was from my nerves growing back from previous surgeries. Then, he decided it was an indication of shingles, which I still don't believe I had. Now, he doesn't know why my ribs are sensitive to touch and hurt. They hurt so much that I cannot lie on them, making sleep very difficult.

I expressed concern to my medical oncologist, and she recommended a bone scan. I'm not sure I want to go for this test just yet. Mentally, I cannot take another major health issue. I don't feel like playing the "what if" game right now.

I had a consult and received insurance approval to have my last surgery. It was scheduled for May 27, 2020. I have met all the qualifications. I am cancer-free, relatively healthy, made the six-month waiting period after radiation, and I am on the surgery schedule. I'm excited yet saddened—

excited that this is the last of the surgeries, but saddened that this will be the last of my boob. Yes, this surgery is to remove the one implant I have left. I'm going to be all natural and have a flat chest. I had so many complications from the implants and don't qualify to have any additional reconstruction procedures. The only two options are to stay lopsided or take the left implant out. I decided to remove the implant. I will be a naturally flat-chested woman. With the correct bra and prosthesis, I can even change sizes. I have a set of small inserts for casual wear and a set of larger ones for those nice, sexy, low V-cut dresses I have. So what size I want to be depends on my mood, the day, and the outfit. May 27, 2020 was my surgery date.

This procedure was relatively simple—so simple and straightforward that it was going to be done in the office and was scheduled for only 30 minutes. Also, I was given only Valium and local anesthesia and had the implant removed. A few sutures, and mom drove me home. The recovery time is just a few days, with very few restrictions. I felt confident about the physician's skill level and hoped for a positive outcome without any further complications.

Right now, I feel good and want to be well. Yes, I still have a few areas of health that need to be addressed, such as my rib pain, my thyroid issue, and my hormone levels, but do I want to know why they are out of range or cause me havoc? I'm not so sure. Some things are better left unknown, right?

I may have a bone scan to figure out my rib issue in July. The pain has been present for more than six months now, so does it matter if I wait another few for the test? In addition, there is always a possibility that the pain is now from bone cancer. It would only make sense since that was the side of my breast cancer. That was also the side that took direct radiation for treatment. Radiation has been known to cause cancer as well. I play the "what if" game quite a bit. It helps me to be realistic and removes some of the shock when the doctor tells me the diagnosis.

I'm not saying that I have bone cancer, but the idea has entered my mind. Hopefully, it is nothing, but at this point, I just don't have the strength or energy to be stressing over this. I'd rather not know.

My thyroid was another issue. The last lab test showed my thyroid was off, and my thyroid antibodies were crazy high. I did have a thyroid ultrasound to check it out, and there was a nodule on my thyroid. A biopsy was recommended. My conservative, smart primary care physician discussed things with me. She gave me a few options, and I asked questions. She gave me options of having a biopsy, going on medication, or waiting and repeating the test in a few months. My thought process was to wait and repeat the test in a few months. We discussed that radiation could have affected my thyroid, and time would bring the lab results down. If the numbers increased, then we would know there was a problem. From there, a repeat ultrasound can be ordered, the nodule reassessed, and, if its larger, a biopsy can be performed. The last step would be medication for the thyroid.

Again, do I want to hear that I can now have thyroid cancer? *No!* Have I thought about it? Of course. Again, let's wait and see. As the saying goes, "time heals all wounds." My primary physician concurred with my decision making.

Hormone levels are my other pending health concern, but I'm not too worried. While my cancer was estrogen- and progesterone-positive, I am not in a hurry to spread my legs for a gynecological visit. I found out this past month that I am not yet in menopause, so the possibility of a hysterectomy is there, especially since I am not taking hormone blocker medications. No thanks. No more surgeries. I'll take my chances. The other option would be taking hormone blocker medication. No thanks. I already had this conversation and don't want to have it again.

And there is the other finding I don't want to know about: ovarian or uterine cancer. I am so over all of this. I don't want any more surgeries, I don't want to take medications, and I don't want to be constantly going to doctor appointments. I hope this is the end of my cancer story. However, my biggest fear is a recurrence.

On June 3, 2020, the recurrence scare came yet again. I developed a large lump on the right side of my chest. Was this a complication from having my left breast implant removed? Was this a new, rapidly growing cancer that decided to show itself? Was this a fluid collection of some sort? What was going on now? The questions started to consume me. The symptoms of this new problem also started to show themselves. Pain, swelling, hardness, difficulty breathing, and difficulty with arm movement were all signs of a major problem.

I told mom about it, and she asked me what I wanted to do about it. I said: "Take me to the ER."

She asked: "When?"

I said, "Now."

Here we go again. Yes, now. If not now, when? In a week? In a month? Yes, now! To the ER I went.

We got to the ER, and only the patient was allowed in due to COVID-19. Mom had to stay in the parking lot until I was seen. She was not happy with that, especially since it was raining. I was taken straight back into the exam room. The nurse started to treat me for cardiac issues when I said I had some shortness of breath. I didn't have cardiac chest pain, I had respiratory issues—chest expansion issues. However, I was hooked up to the EKG. I was given aspirin and oxygen, an IV was placed, labs were drawn, and I had the COVID swab test, all prior to the doctor seeing me.

When the doctor examined me, his first thought was I had a muscle pull that was protruding and causing this hard, large lump on my chest. I was given a muscle relaxant, but it didn't help with the swelling or pain. Next, a CT was ordered to rule out fluid collection or lung problems. When the results came back, they showed a right breast implant rupture. Hmm, can't be. I didn't have an implant on that side and hadn't for a year. I had to prove to the doctor with my previous CT report that I didn't have an implant there. He then called the radiologist to have the report reread.

The final conclusion was that I had a collection of fluid in my chest. Now, what type of fluid was it? Where did it come from? What caused this to happen?

I texted mom and told her to go home, as she was still waiting in the parking lot. I told her most likely I would be admitted to the hospital for this to be fixed. That is what happened. This hospital admission was the worse one yet. While I had to wait hours again for the transport, no visitors were allowed in the hospital due to COVID-19.

How long would I be I the hospital? What was wrong with me? I spent the night in the hospital with nothing to do, no one to talk to, and a list of questions. When morning came, I was actually scheduled to have this fluid area drained. Down to the procedural suite I went. The doctor told me I would only have local anesthetic and the type of fluid that came out of me would determine what the diagnosis would be. Anxiously, I sat on the exam table and prepared for the procedure.

The doctor proceeded to push a needle into my chest and drew out reddish fluid that looked like blood to me. The total collection was just about a liter of fluid. I felt better now that the lump was just about flat. I had chest expansion again, and the pain was minimal. I was fixed! Now, why did this happen? What type of fluid was it? What did this all mean? Back to my private and lonely hospital room to wait for pathology results and write down more questions.

When I awoke in the morning, the drained and flattened site was again raised and filled with fluid. I told the nurse, and another ultrasound was performed. Yes, more fluid had accumulated. Where was the fluid coming from? Did this area need to be drained again? Did I have a leaking blood vessel? How many more days would I have to be here? All were valid questions, but there were no answers and no actions were being taken.

I wanted action, answers, to be fixed, and discharged. It had been four days and nothing was being done—no second drainage, no vessel studies, no pathology reports, no visitors, no nothing. I was confined to my room, and that was it.

I had to do something. I decided to call my breast doctor in Tampa and told her what happened. She told me to drive over there when I get discharged and go to urgent care. She would have all the orders waiting for me. I discussed my situation with the hospitalist and decided that discharge would be best. I had been in the local hospital for four days and was right back where I started, with a fluid-filled lump, pain, swelling, and lack of chest expansion.

From discharge, I drove four hours across the state to Tampa. My chest was hurting, and I was in extreme pain, but I felt this was my only option. I went to the urgent care center my breast surgeon had suggested. This 28-bed urgent care, with room sizes bigger than a hotel room was impressive. As soon as I stated my name, I saw the doctor. Again, EKG, IV, labs, and a CT scan all were done in an hour. With the results of the scan, I was scheduled for another drainage of my chest. Five hundred milliliters of fluid were removed. I was impressed. I had been in the local hospital for four days, and this specialty urgent care not only repeated everything but drained me in four hours! Driving four hours was so worth it to me to receive high-quality care. It is just a shame that a four-hour drive was needed. Why are the doctors in my area such dumbasses?

In addition, these doctors left a drain in me, so if more fluid were to accumulate again, I wouldn't need to have the procedure again. *Smart!* I saw the breast surgeon at 8 a.m. the next morning. She went over the lab results and told me it was not cancer, it was not a vessel leak, and not trauma related. All good news. She did order an MRI and PET scan for two weeks later, when the drain was removed. This was all coming together. She told me to call with any issues or problems between now and then. Why couldn't my local hospital tell me this and arrange for these procedures?

When the drain came out two weeks later, the MRI and PET scan were completed. The breast surgeon telephoned the results to me within two hours of the exam being completed. Tests revealed thoracic lymph nodes and areas of concern in the lungs. A repeat for follow-up in three to six months was recommended. Basically, these were all things I already had known. All follow-up diagnostic tests would be performed in Tampa for continuity of care, evaluation of reports by highly qualified specialty physicians, and fast turnaround times.

Recurrence Concerns

I would question the treatment if, in a year, the cancer is back. If for some reason my cancer should return shortly, my decision is to do nothing. How many times can I go through this? To me it means give up already, my body is meant to have cancer. I have already prolonged my life by three to five years, which is the typical time from initial onset to death from cancer. The five-year window is the key. If a person can make five years of being cancer-free, their cancer usually does not return, and they are "clear." Notice that I did not use the "C word," cured. I said *cleared*. Medical oncologists do not like the word "cured," but "clear" and "remission" are fine.

There is always a chance for recurrence, something I have already thought about. Quality versus quantity of life—that is the discussion. I for one would rather have quality than quantity. I do not want to go through chemo again, and deal with all the side effects of nausea, loss of appetite, fatigue, low immunity, being chained to the doctor's office, or worry about radiation daily. I want to feel well, be free, come and go as I please, meet people for lunch, go shopping, and travel without worries.

If I should become terminal in the near future, I just want to know two things: First that I am terminal, and second, how many months I have to live. Why do I want to know this? There are several reasons. I need to ensure all my wishes are carried out as I had previously planned. This is the time to answer any questions people have about my will and trust before I die, so they know what to do when my time is up. I want to travel and see a few more places before I am not longer able to do so. I don't care if I should die while traveling, either. I have an insurance plan to cover me. One phone call and everything is prearranged, from my flight home in a box to my cremation instructions.

Finally, I want to plan and host my "goodbye party." I have thought of this, too. Crazy or a great idea? Why not? It will be a three-day weekend, open-house, party-style event where people can come and pay their respects, and we can say our final goodbyes. People can share stories, we will have games, drinks, food, and pictures, with a heavenly backdrop that they can have as a souvenir. I will also give out party favors (small dove ornaments) as keepsakes. I will also publicly give away my previously assigned personal items. No sense in waiting for me to die. Take them while I'm on my deathbed—that is better. Can you tell that I have previously planned this party? This only works if I'm terminal and a timeline is known. Hopefully, the natural progression of death will take place, and I will not need to plan this party.

Final Thoughts

In this book, I believe I have given the reader a unique look at my breast cancer experiences and a different perspective on some of the problems that may arise during their journey. I have provided the reader with an inside look at my own personal story. I have provided factual information about breast cancer and have exposed areas of concern that doctors may not completely explain to patients.

I hope that you have found my story beneficial, in case you come across a dumbass doctor as well. Dumbass doctors can be found anywhere. This book can serve as a guide to know the truths about the cancer modalities, inspire one to think about the steps they want to take if a traumatic event occurs in your life, and allow you to make the proper decisions, whether you are a patient or caregiver.

Special Thanks

A special thank-you to my loving mother, Maria Errante-Parrino, who sketched the cover in pencil for this book. I am thankful she designed it with my vision in mind.

Thank you to my editors Katie Cline and Bill Bowers, whose professionalism and hard work were instrumental in the completion of this project.

References

1. Riter, B. April 20, 2012. "Does Cancer Hurt?" Retrieved April 3, 2019 from Cancer Resource Center of the Finger Lakes. http://www.crcfl.net/index.php/does-cancer-hurt-2/

2. National Cancer Institute https://www.cancer.gov/

3. M. D. Anderson Cancer Center https://www.mdanderson.org/patients-family/diagnosis-treatment.html

4. Eldridge, L. 2018. "Does Cancer Hurt?" Retrieved April 3, 2019 from https://www.verywellhealth.com/does-cancer-hurt-2249010

5. CancerCare.org. 2019. "Coping with Cancer-related Weight Changes and Muscle Loss." Retrieved April 21, 2019 from https://www.cancercare.org/publications/140-coping_with_cancer-related_weight_changes_and_muscle_loss

6. Garcia, S. 2019. "The Dangers of Dr. Google." Retrieved April 23, 2019 from https://moffitt.org/take-charge/take-charge-story-archive/the-dangers-of-doctor-google/?source=dg

7. American Cancer Society Medical and Editorial Content Team. "Managing Nutrition During Cancer and Treatment." Chemocare. Retrieved April 25, 2019 from http://www.chemocare.com/chemotherapy/health-wellness/managing-nutrition-during-cancer-and-treatment.aspx

8. Benefits of good nutrition during cancer treatment. American Cancer Society. Retrieved on April 25, 2019 from https://www.cancer.org/treatment/survivorship-during-and-after-treatment/staying-active/nutrition/nutrition-during-treatment/benefits.html

9. Exercising during chemotherapy for breast or colon cancer has long-term benefits. American Society of Clinical Oncology. Retrieved April 25, 2019 from

https://www.asco.org/about-asco/press-center/news-releases/exercising-during-chemotherapy-breast-or-colon-cancer-has-long

10. Exercises after breast cancer surgery. American Cancer Society. Retrieved April 25, 2019 from https://www.cancer.org/cancer/breast-cancer/treatment/surgery-for-breast-cancer/exercises-after-breast-cancer-surgery.html

11. Stephan, P. 2019. "What is the Cancer Antigen 27.29 Test? Tumor marker test used to monitor metastatic breast cancer." Retrieved June 30, 2019 from https://www.verywellhealth.com/cancer-antigen-2729-430607

12. "Radiation Therapy for Breast Cancer." Mayo Foundation for Medical Education. Retrieved July 16, 2019 from https://www.mayoclinic.org/tests-procedures/radiation-therapy-for-breast-cancer/about/pac-20384940

13. Intensity Modulated Radiation Therapy (IMRT). 2019. MayoClinic. Retrieved September 11, 2019 from https://www.mayoclinic.org/tests-procedures/intensity-modulated-radiation-therapy/about/pac-20385147

14. Intensity Modulated Radiation Therapy. May 2019. Retrieved September 11, 2019 from https://www.radiologyinfo.org/en/info.cfm?pg=imrt#therapy-overview

15. UPMC Hillman Cancer Center. 2019. Retrieved November 21, 2019 from https://hillman.upmc.com/cancer-care/radiation-oncology/treatment/external-beam/3d-conformal

16. Five things you need to know about ports. Retrieved April 11, 2020 from https://www.healthline.com/health/breast-cancer/rethink-bc-ports#1

17. Breastcancer.org. Retrieved April 20, 2020 from https://www.breastcancer.org/treatment/druglist/tamoxifen

18. "Vagal Maneuvers for a Fast Heart Rate". WebMD. March 12, 2014. Retrieved April 20, 2020.

19. Rxlist.com. https://www.rxlist.com/arimidex-drug.htm. Retrieved on April 20, 2020.

20. National Cancer Institute. Retrieved May 11, 2020 from https://www.cancer.gov/publications/dictionaries/cancer-terms/def/patient-advocate